**Some Samples From
The Sampler—**

- What vitamin supplements you need—and why.
  (Chapter II)
- What to feed—and when not to feed—your pre-school child.
  (Chapter X)
- How to "mine" valuable minerals—in your own body!
  (Chapter IV)
- Honey, oatmeal, cream—not for breakfast but for a rejuvenating facial treatment.
  (Chapter VI)
- Your body's control center and how it works.
  (Chapter IX)

Your own health is one of the most important concerns in your life. Learn more about the *natural* way to good health from these leading writers and experienced authorities in

Your Natural Health Sampler

Your Natural Health Sampler

THE BEST OF TODAY'S WRITING ON HEALTH, NUTRITION, DIET AND BEAUTY

Keats Publishing, Inc.   New Canaan, Connecticut

Acknowledgement is made to the following for their kind permission to include material which appears in this book:

What You Should Know About Proteins has been excerpted from YOUR HEALTH IS WHAT YOU MAKE IT by C. W. Whitmoyer, Sr., D.Sc. (Cloth, $10.00), an Exposition-Banner book, published by Exposition Press, Jericho, New York.

Minerals: The Mine Within You has been excerpted from COMMON SENSE NUTRITION by Ruth Little Carey, Ph.D., Irma Bachmann Vyhmeister, M.S., and Jennie Stagg Hudson, M.A. (Paperback, $2.95), published by Pacific Press Publishing Association, Mountain View, California.

Other chapters have been excerpted from books and magazines published by Keats Publishing, Inc.

YOUR NATURAL HEALTH SAMPLER

Pivot Edition published 1973

Copyright © 1973 by Keats Publishing, Inc.

Printed in the United States of America

Library of Congress Catalog Card Number: 73-80031

Pivot Health Books are published by Keats Publishing, Inc.
212 Elm Street, New Canaan, Connecticut 06840

TABLE OF CONTENTS

ABOUT THE AUTHORS

LINDA CLARK, eminent researcher/reporter in the fields of nutrition, beauty and health, is in constant touch with the public through her column in *Let's Live* Magazine, as well as through her books. Her concern is with man's well-being, how he looks, feels and thinks. The key words in her philosophy are balance, sensibility and completeness. In this total view of health Linda Clark considers everything from cooking utensils, to mental attitudes, to beauty . . . since health is the first step to looking well. We must not correct the flaws in our bodies by covering them up, but by a change of diet and proper exercise; not by miracles but by sensible, health-conscious, natural living.

RUTH LITTLE CAREY, PhD, IRMA BACHMANN VYHMEISTER, MS, AND JENNIE STAGG HUDSON, MA, are all authors who are also professors of nutrition, and who have undertaken the task of translating the scientific jargon of research and nutritional data into a form more understandable to the layman. Skilled at selection and condensation, they offer the public a complete overall view of healthful nutritional living.

BEATRICE TRUM HUNTER is a highly respected leader in the natural foods field. A scholarly, conscientious writer, she received an award from the Friends of Nature in 1960 for her work in educating the public in the hazards of pesticides. Besides Mrs. Hunter's much-acclaimed books, she has given demonstrations in whole-grain bread making, lectures, and has made radio and TV appearances. Her cookbooks explode any myth that what is good for you has to taste bad. Her recipes are easy, delicious! and scrupulously nutritious. And she can be applauded by everyone for helping to revive the tradition of wholesome, wonderful, home-baked bread.

GENA LARSON pioneered the use of sound nutrition principles in school lunch programs while managing the cafeteria at Helix High School, La Mesa, California. This program and its spectacular results have influenced cafeteria programs in many schools and colleges throughout the country. A teacher and lecturer, Mrs. Larson's approach to nutrition is clear and uncomplicated. She gives a much-needed emphasis to pre-natal, and to the early years of a baby's life. She also gives special attention to the health of the mother, knowing that a sound body can be produced only through another sound body. Gena Larson includes the entire family in her picture of healthful living. She is a good guide through today's labyrinth of nutritional politics.

FRIEDA NUSZ arranges a happy combination of wholesome naturalness and modern technology in her *Natural Foods Blender Cookbook*. Sympathetic to today's needs for speed and convenience, she has devised a plan which is entirely suitable to a twentieth century tempo—without the forfeiture of health! Usually convenient food means empty food. But Frieda Nusz has pointed a nutritious way out of this dilemma.

PAGE and ABRAMS. Dr. Page is head of the famed Page Clinic in St. Petersburg Beach, Florida. After forty years of clinical observation, testing and treatment, he developed a basic program, putting it in print with H. Leon Abrams, for capturing good health. Taking body measurements and detailed endocrine and blood tests, Dr. Page can diagnose the body's problem, and prescribe correction. Good health is achieved, not through more and more drugs, but by a change in diet. His devotion to the science of body chemistry and his interest in nutrition has led Dr. Page to the development of a total, natural health program.

VIRGINIA CASTLETON THOMAS, beauty editor of *Prevention Magazine*, really understands the attainment of beauty through nature. You can see it in her face, and in anyone who uses the surprisingly simple formulas that she writes about. Again, we have sensibility and sympathy with today's needs of wholesomeness and convenience. Using ordinary foods that are staples in our homes, such as cider vinegar, honey or eggs, she teaches us to look and feel better. Her concepts are based on sound principles, on her knowledge of the acid/base balance of our skin, and of vitamins. We achieve a healthful harmony and well-being by feeding our skin and hair from the outside as well as internally. This kind of beauty is simply external nutrition.

CARLSON WADE is a responsible researcher, as well as a writer and editor in the nutritional and natural foods field. He often undertakes the laborious work of tracking down and assimilating the reports, analyses, experiments and all the various findings that are being made . . . making them available to the public in a more comprehensible form. He keeps us oriented in this ever-changing and growing field of health.

MAX WARMBRAND, one of the few practising naturopaths, is also an osteopath and chiropractor, and of course "down to earth". His approach to health is totally basic and essential relying on a pure, wholesome and discriminatory view of food. He knows both how sickness can be avoided, and as a doctor, how the body can be restored and re-built through eating closer to nature. However, his true credit should come from the countless people who have regained their health through his programs and care. He has been practising medicine for fifty years, and is co-founder of the accredited Florida Spa in Orlando.

C. W. WHITMOYER is also a doctor very much concerned with health preservation, as well as health restoration. As a biochemist and scientist he reminds us that maintaining the health of our minds and bodies is our responsibility, and also that this maintenance is based on scientific principles. His subjects range from the more technical aspects of vitamins, minerals and cholesterol, to health problems in a more social context such as "Drugs and Health" or "Stress and Health". He emphasizes what we all tend to avoid thinking about: that we must gain control of our health through knowledge of our bodies and the way they work for us.

PUBLISHER'S INTRODUCTION

To be concerned about our health, to try to attune our eating and living habits to the precepts of health, is not to be involved in fads or lost causes. Rather, it is urgent that we begin to listen to some of the fine researchers, doctors and writers in the fields of nutrition and natural foods. Our environment becomes more threatening to our health every day—an increased awareness of our bodies and their functioning is not the solution to the problem, but it is one of the many steps that we should be taking, in order to continue living on this planet.

But it is not only this, very real, necessity that drives us to an interest in wholesome food and natural living. It is the pleasure and satisfaction that comes from home-baked bread, beautiful skin, renewed vigor and a general feeling of well-being. The causes that press us to be more knowledgeable about vitamins, body chemistry or food values are doleful and forbidding. The result is happy, for we are rediscovering vitality.

Pre-prepared foods are out . . . nutritious, fresh foods are a delightful new in. Hormone imbalance and body disfunction are out . . . regained balance, comfort and physical effectiveness are in. Convenience and speed, based on loss, are out . . . fun and ease, with heightened nutrition, are in!

We confess that this book is a teaser. It offers only a sampling of what is available—drawing from several different areas of nutrition and natural living. It is, itself, only an introduction.

Each of the authors in this book is respected and enlightened. The sum of what they write about is of utmost importance to our survival.

ONE

NOTES FOR
THE NOVICE BREADMAKER

by

BEATRICE TRUM HUNTER

> **—Beatrice Trum Hunter's
> Whole-Grain Baking Sampler**

REVOLT against plastic food in a plastic culture is in full swing, and commercial white bread has become the target for justified spoofing. It has been dubbed as "pre-sliced absorbent cotton," "cotton fluff wrapped up in a skin," and "pappy, tasteless, soft, aerated substances that are as appetizing as white foam rubber without the spring and the bounce." One writer commented that our bread is sliced, wrapped, steamed, and whitened to duplicate the consistency of old newspapers, with an unforgettable aroma of nothingness.

There is a campus revolt, with students demanding "honest" whole-grain breads in the school cafeterias. There is supermarket revolt, with housewives demanding an end to overpriced deceptive "balloon bread" that is blown up to monstrous proportions. There is consumer revolt, with many concerned about the hazards of artificial emulsifiers, texturizers, stabilizers, dyes, mold retarders, and a host of other chemical adjuncts permitted in commercial baking. There is more consumer revolt, revealed when much of the bread served in restaurants, airplanes, hospitals, and other public places is rejected and ultimately finds its way to the pig farms.

"Who should make bread?" asked Sylvester Graham, that social critic whose name became associated with flour and crackers. In 1837, Graham demonstrated that neither the public bakers nor domestic servants had "those sensibilities and affections which alone can secure that careful attention, that soundness of judgment, that accuracy of operation, without which the best of bread cannot even uniformly, if ever, be produced."

With the flowery embellishments of the times, Graham concluded:

"It is the wife, the mother only—she who loves her husband and her children as women ought to love, and who rightly perceives the relations between the dietetic habits and physical and moral condition of her loved ones, and justly appreciates the importance of good

3

bread to their physical and moral welfare—she alone it is, who will be ever inspired by that cordial and unremitting affection and solicitude which will excite the vigilance, secure the attention, and prompt the action requisite to success, and essential to the attainment of that maturity of judgment and skillfulness of operation, which are the indispensable attributes of a perfect breadmaker. And could wives and mothers fully comprehend the importance of good bread in relation to all the bodily and intellectual and moral interests of their husbands and children, and in relation to the domestic and social and civil welfare of mankind, and to their religious prosperity, both for time and eternity, they would estimate the art and duty of breadmaking far, very far more highly than they now do. They would then realize that, as no one can feel so deep and delicate an interest for their husbands' and children's happiness as they do, so no one can be so proper a person to prepare for them that portion of their aliment, which requires a degree of care and attention that can only spring from the lively affections and solicitude of a wife and mother."

Although Graham advised that the art of bread baking be returned to the wife and mother, today bread is being made by men as well as women, from teenagers to octogenarians. Many individuals have returned to the art of bread baking. Others approach it as novices. Many would bake bread, if only given a little encouragement and instruction. Thus, this sampler meets a need. All who make bread admit enthusiastically that bread baking is a creative, satisfying experience. It gets down to the essentials in life.

Only a few simple techniques need to be learned. Ingredients are readily available. No special equipment is necessary. Nor is breadmaking time-consuming. Some breads can be made, from start to finish, in less than two hours. There are breads that require no kneading—a practice long viewed as synonymous with drudgery.

While no *one* bread may satisfy all palates, there is variety enough for everyone to find some breads to his liking. The world seems to be divided into two groups: those who favor light-colored, feathery breads, contrasted to those who enjoy the dark-colored, dense ones. Perhaps it is habit. Perhaps it is social custom, of patricians versus plebeians. In this sampler, you will find breads both light and dark, spongy and hearty.

In general, I have eliminated from consideration those breads dependent on devitalized flours. The milling of wheat into refined white flour removes, among other nutrients:

    60 per cent of the calcium
    71 per cent of the phosphorus
    85 per cent of the magnesium
    77 per cent of the potassium
    78 per cent of the sodium

In addition to these major elements, many trace elements also essential for life and health are removed:

    40 per cent of the chromium
    86 per cent of the manganese
    76 per cent of the iron
    89 per cent of the cobalt
    68 per cent of the copper
    78 per cent of the zinc
    48 per cent of the molybdenum

In "enriched" flour, only the calcium and iron are put back, and the iron is added in a form poorly absorbed. Despite the "enrichment" program, the country continues to show signs of calcium and iron deficiencies.

In some recipes that follow, where white flour is used to a limited extent, it is *unbleached,* and fortified with the Triple Rich Cornell Formula, which adds wheat germ, soy flour, and nonfat dry milk powder. These three ingredients raise the nutritional standards of the flour, without radically changing either the taste or appearance of the finished baked product.

For many recipes, I have specified dry yeast granules, instead of compressed yeast cakes or packages of yeast. The yeast cakes, with limited shelf life, and requiring refrigeration, now contain an undesirable added antioxidant. The major cost of the dry yeast granules packed in individual packages consists mainly of the packaging material. For thrift, and to avoid the objectionable antioxidant, it is wise to purchase the dry yeast granules loose, by the pound, half pound, or quarter pound. The loose dry yeast granules are readily found in health food stores or through mail order companies. This yeast should be transferred to a tightly closed container. Stored in a cool, dry place, it will remain active, if unrefrigerated, for at least six months. For anyone who bakes regularly, buying the dry yeast granules in quantity assures a supply on hand for each baking.

One tablespoonful of the granules equals one package of dry yeast granules, or one cake of compressed yeast. One pound of dry yeast granules contains approximately forty-eight tablespoons. If you wish to convert a traditional recipe, and it calls for one ounce of yeast, use three tablespoons of the dry yeast granules.

For the beginning bread baker, the *only* crucial act in the entire procedure is at the beginning: softening the yeast. It is vital to have the water at the proper temperature in order to activate the yeast. The water should be *warm; not* hot; *not* lukewarm. Hot water will kill the yeast and inactivate it. Lukewarm water is too cool and fails to activate the yeast. If the mixture does not bubble within five to ten minutes after the yeast has been softened in the warm water, the water was probably too hot, or not warm enough. Start anew, with fresh yeast and water. Otherwise, you will waste precious bread ingredients and have bricklike loaves. If, on your second try, you have been careful to have the water at the proper temperature, but still fail to activate the yeast, assume that the yeast is too old and has become inactive. Replace it with fresh stock.

A small amount of sweetening added to the warm water and yeast will hasten the action of the yeast. However, be careful not to add *cold* honey or molasses in any quantity to the water-yeast mixture, or it will retard, rather than hasten the action. Potato water, which not only helps to keep bread moist, also hastens the rising.

If you are pressed for time during a baking session, use more baking yeast. If you double the amount, it will not affect the quality of the bread, and it will shorten the rising time.

Breads made with yeast keep fresh longer, and do not dry out as quickly as those made with baking powder. Yeast is rich in the B vitamins, while baking powders are B-vitamin destroyers.

In an attempt to substitute liquid vegetable oils for solid fats as much as possible in food preparation, I extended this procedure to bread baking as well. Not only is it healthier, by reducing the intake of saturated fats, but it is *easier*. It is far quicker to measure liquid oil than the cumbersome water-displacement or actual measurement of solid fats. Also, remember to measure the oil *before* you measure your honey, molasses, or other syrupy sweeteners. The cup, being coated with oil, will allow the sweetener to leave the cup readily. None gets wasted.

Which vegetable oils are suitable for bread baking? Any of the mild-flavored ones (corn, peanut, safflower, sesame, etc.) are good. Avoid the strong-flavored ones, which may be fine for salad dressing, or for brushing over fish to be baked, but will overpower baked products.

My own experience has been that the most satisfactory way of greasing bread pans and muffin pans is to use butter. Oil is less satisfactory for these utensils. It makes the baked products stick, and difficult to remove. On the other hand, cooky sheets, and mixing bowls for storing balls of dough while rising, are satisfactorily greased with oil.

Just as bleached, refined flours should be shunned because of their nutritional impoverishment, so should refined sugars be avoided. Fortunately, there are nutritionally rich natural sweeteners that can be substituted. Honey is perhaps the first choice, in popularity. Choose the light-flavored ones for baking (for example, clover) so that they do not predominate in the baked product. The dark-flavored ones (for example, buckwheat) are good on toast, waffles, etc.

Honey is especially favored for baking since it retains moisture. This keeps baked products from drying out.

Unsulfured molasses, stronger in flavor than honey, is excellent for certain types of baked products. Blackstrap molasses, nutritionally very rich, is somewhat bitter, and must be used sparingly. It is good in combination with unsulfured molasses or with honey.

What other natural sweeteners can be used? Maple syrup and maple sugar are delicate in flavor. Sorghum molasses, malt, and carob syrups all have distinctive flavors. They appear slightly less sweet than either honey or molasses.

There are still other natural sweeteners. Carob powder, malted-milk powder, whey powder, and nonfat dry milk powder all have a natural sweetness. The use of dried fruits, carrots, and squash can add sweetness to baked products, and allows the cook to cut down on other sweetening agents in the recipes.

For the beginning breadmaker, the entire procedure of kneading seems like some skillful art. It really isn't! Here are a few hints. When the flour and liquid are well mixed in the bowl, and no longer stick to the sides, the dough is ready to be turned out and kneaded.

"How do you knead?" When a young woman asked me this question, I was stunned. But anyone knows how to knead! I began to mull it over. I grew up in an age when everyone's mother or grandmother made homemade bread. I learned how to knead by watching. Young people today may not have this opportunity. So, for those who have never seen anyone knead, this is the closest description I can give. Flour your fingers and palms and handle the dough lightly. Fold the edges of the dough toward the center, press down, and away, with your palms. Turn the dough over, and repeat. Continue doing this, quite rhythmically, until the dough is "smooth and elastic." You will know when the dough has reached this stage—which may take five minutes, eight minutes, ten minutes, or even fifteen minutes—when the dough no longer sticks to your hands or the board. If you press it with your finger, it will spring back into shape. Avoid overkneading, which may injure the baking quality of the gluten, and result in poor texture and volume. After you finish kneading, oil the surface of the dough. This will prevent it from drying out or cracking as it rises.

The gluten may also be injured if it is allowed to stand too long before being punched down. If the dough is allowed to rise too high in the pans before baking, it will result in coarse-grained bread. On the other hand, if you do not allow the dough to rise sufficiently in the pans before baking, your bread will be as heavy as a brick. All of this sounds more complicated than it is. A little experience will teach you how long to knead, and how long to allow the dough to rise.

How do you shape the dough for bread pan form? This is another question often asked. Divide your dough evenly into the number of loaves you intend to bake. Press, or roll, each piece into a flat, oblong piece. Take one long side, and fold one third of the dough over, and press it with the palm of your hand to seal.

Then fold the other long side, overlapping the first. Press, and seal, as before. From the end, fold one third of the dough over. Press and seal. Fold the other end, overlapping the first. Press and seal. You have made an envelope. Now roll the sheet of dough lengthwise, like a jelly roll, making a round, compact loaf. Seal the overlap, and place the dough in a greased bread pan, with the overlap underneath.

The loaf should be half the depth of the pan. After the dough rises, the sides of the dough should be near the top of the pan, and the center should be well rounded.

Certain types of breads bake well when there is steam in the oven. You can place a pan of hot water on the bottom rack, while the bread is being baked.

If you like a shiny crust on bread, brush it with a beaten egg yolk, mixed with one tablespoon of cold water or milk, before you bake the bread. If you like to decorate your breads with seeds, brush the tops of the bread with this same mixture, before sprinkling the seeds on top. They will stay more securely in place. If you like hard-crusted breads, allow air to circulate around the loaves when they cool. If you enjoy soft-crusted breads, wrap the loaves in cloths while they are cooling. Or, you can brush the tops with melted butter, water, or milk, when you take the loaves out of the oven.

In most instances, quantities used in the following recipes yield more than a single loaf of bread. Usually pressed for time, I dislike wasting it. It is just as easy to make a few loaves of bread at one time as it is to make a single loaf. If you make a quantity beyond your own immediate needs, you will find that homemade bread is a much appreciated present to other. It also freezes well. If you have no friends (unlikely) or if you lack a freezer, you can always divide the recipe in half. If you think that you can't make a large batch because you lack the strength, think again. You can always mix a large amount in two bowls, or divide the dough in half, and knead each half individually. Some people have told me that they could not make homemade bread because they lacked large mixing bowls. What an excuse! A large enameled washbasin, a new scrubbing pail, or a vessel used for canning, all can double as mixing bowls.

If you plan to mix or knead stiff doughs, work at a low table in the kitchen, so that your arms are not bent awkwardly at a fatiguing angle. If you don't have a low table, try placing your mixing bowl in the bottom of the kitchen sink. If your bowl is too large to fit into the sink, instead of trying to lower the bowl, you can raise yourself. Place your bowl on the counter top, and you stand on a low footstool.

There is an elemental joy in baking bread. Many people like to get their hands into the dough. Perhaps we are still children playing with mud pies. Some persons especially enjoy working with yeast dough, which seems to have a life of its own, as it rises, falls, and rises again. I've even heard some exclaim as the bread comes out of the oven, "Such beautiful babies!" And who hasn't enjoyed the experience of various bread fragrances? The pungent aroma of fermented sourdough, the yeasty smell of the bread sponge, and the redolence wafting from the oven, as the bread is being baked? I shall say no more. Both author and reader are drooling.

Does homemade bread keep well? My husband's stock answer is, "No, not in this household. It's eaten up too quickly to spoil." Since homemade bread does not have the mold retarders of calcium or sodium propionate, used by most commercial bakers, it is best to keep bread refrigerated. This is especially true in hot, humid weather. Whole grain breads are more perishable than those made from refined flours. But even the whole grain ones will keep for one to two weeks, if refrigerated.

Many of the bread recipes have free-form shapes

of round loaves or long loaves, without the use of bread pans. There is a creative sense in "doing your own thing." You can form whatever shape you wish. You can decorate the tops of breads with seeds, pattern them with crisscross knife slashes, make them shine by brushing them with beaten egg yolk, or give them whatever other finishing touches you wish with your own special signature. Perhaps the free-form loaf is but another aspect of the revolt against the mechanization of life. The bread pans make for uniformity, the free form expresses a handiwork. Enough said. Begin to bake bread.

TWO

HOW MANY VITAMINS
SHOULD YOU TAKE?

by

LINDA CLARK

—Health Today magazine

I AM ASKED again and again, "What vitamins should I take, and how many?" The answer is: nobody knows. Except you. Why? There are several reasons.

1. Roger J. Williams, Ph.D., who is professor of the Department of Biochemistry, University of Texas, as well as the discoverer of the B vitamin, pantothenic acid, states that because there is such a great variety of individual differences, no single rule applies to everyone. For example, no one has the same finger prints. But the differences do not stop here. Anatomy books show pictures of hearts and other organs of many people. None are alike in size, shape, even often in location! Obviously, if these organs are different in appearance, they may also work differently. So you cannot generalize on a *physical* basis that you need the same kind and amount of nutrients as your friends, your neighbors or even the members of your family. Take vitamin A as an example.

In 1932 Mead Johnson offered $15,000 as an award to anyone who could find out how much vitamin A a person needs. There were no takers and after 13 years the offer was withdrawn. One man in England was reported by Dr. Williams as being healthy on no vitamin A at all; and a woman in Pittsburgh, whose doctor prescribed 50,000 I.U. daily, was also apparently healthy. Many nutritionists usually settle for 25,000 international units per day, but that may or may not be the right amount for you.

2. Besides physical differences, each person possesses different genes. If your forefathers were Scandinavian, or Italian, or Oriental, your *inherited needs* differ. Each race thrives on food indigenous to that country. The Scandinavians, with cold winters and short growing seasons thrive on fish. Italians, with a sunny climate and long growing seasons thrive on fresh fruits and vegetables. Orientals subsist mainly on white rice, a diet which would produce for Americans beriberi, a B vitamin deficiency disease, since the B vita-

min coating is removed from white rice and Americans do not get vitamin B, usually, in large enough amounts to compensate for this loss. (Orientals probably do.) So look to your ancestors and their many centuries of eating certain foods which may have conditioned your genes, thus *your* preferences for certain foods, which may turn other people off.

3. What about your *temperament?* Are you the emotional type or calm as a cucumber? If you are highly nervous, and/or an insomniac, it stands to reason that you are going to need more of the soothing foods such as B complex and calcium, than your more phlegmatic friends and relatives. There is little need for them to load up on such nutrients if they have no use for them in high amounts. But you may need more.

4. What is your *occupation,* or way of life? Is it sedentary or physically active? Do you walk to work or ride? Dr. Jean Mayer, nutritionist of Harvard University, is convinced that the amount of exercise you take determines the amount of food you should eat. Less active people, he believes, need less food, otherwise they store the excess as fat. More active people spend more physical energy, need more food and use up their fuel faster; they are rarely fat. Even the stress of a sedentary executive determines the amount of fuel he burns, whereas a relaxed secretary, also sedentary, may need far less than her high-strung boss.

Your size and frame is another clue. Usually a large-framed, active man may need more food than a tiny less active woman, but not always. I know a couple in which the wife is a perfect size 8 and her husband, who has a football build, has been more than 50 pounds overweight. They both eat the same menu but she eats more than he does! A doctor spotted the cause: the difference between these two was poor assimilation, or metabolism, in the man. When the doctor put him on a diet best for *him,* he lost 45 pounds in two months, feels wonderful and had to get a complete set of new clothes.

5. *What kind of food do you eat?* A farmer who is raising his own organic food, natural dairy products and other goodies, is certainly not going to need the extra vitamins as do city folks who eat refined and processed foods. Our great grandparents ate whole natural food, got plenty of exercise and never heard of vitamins. Today, people deprived of these whole foods need supplements as insurance to fill in the gaps of the missing nutrients.

There are few common denominators for everybody. Those who pride themselves because they have regular injections of B_{12}, or take a dollop of a single vitamin, are kidding themselves. Nature does not work that way! *In natural food all vitamins and minerals are present.* At least 60 nutrients are needed by everyone, every day of your life. Witness the birth defects, now confirmed by scientists as resulting from a pregnant woman eating a one-sided diet. Such a diet may take longer to play havoc with grown adults, but sooner or later it catches up with them, too.

Every known and unknown vitamin and mineral is needed. The best way to get these is in whole natural foods and supplements. Synthetics do not contain them all. Synthetics have their place in temporary treatment for a diseased state, but nutritional doctors feel that taken in high amounts, too long, can become the equivalent of whipping a tired horse. Natural vitamins are nothing more than concentrated food. If you must make a choice, choose whole food first, supplements second. In food, variety is imperative too. To get everything, one doctor has advised people to eat a different menu each day of the month. Too many people get into a rut and eat hamburgers and french fries every day. Buy yourself some paperback health-gourmet cookbooks at the health store and stretch your eating horizons. It's fun.

How do you find out what and how much you need? First, analyze your needs, as I have outlined. Next, improve your over-all eating and wait and see how you feel after a fair trial. Then, very slowly, start on supplements, at first in *small amounts*. Use the trial and error method. Watch out for allergies. Many people are allergic to wheat products and their by-products. A very few cannot take even natural vitamin C. A friend of mine breaks out in a rash from eating the wonderful, native fruits when she is in Hawaii. You need not become a hypochondriac; just be intelligent until you learn what is the best program for *you*. By the way, there is no capsule large enough to hold all these 60 nutrients in natural form.

If you can find a nutritional doctor to help you, grab him; he is rare. If you can't, no one in the world can dictate to you what to eat. You know yourself and your reactions even better than a doctor who does not know you. So, through self-discovery you *can* find the kind and amount of vitamins you need. Try it!

THREE

WHAT YOU SHOULD KNOW ABOUT PROTEINS

by

C. W. WHITMOYER

—Your Health Is What You Make It

ALL NUTRIENTS required by the human or animal system are of great importance. But the proteins do occupy the center of the stage. This is so partly because such a large percentage of the composition of dry matter in the body consists of proteins; partly because protein is such an essential material in many of the chemical processes of the body; and partly because it is constantly destroyed by the activities of the body.

The name of the substance we know as proteins was originated by the Swedish chemist Berzelius in the eighteenth century. It was derived from the Greek word *protein,* which means of the first rank. Because of the great importance, the many functions, and the vast diversity of types of molecules tailored precisely to perform a variety of tasks, the proteins certainly qualify as being of first rank.

Proteins are present in plants as a result of chemical reactions which take place subsequent to the photosynthetic process by which carbon dioxide and water were converted to carbohydrates. In plants the proteins are found in the most concentrated form in the seeds, such as the bean or the kernel of wheat or corn. The area of the germ of the seed is especially rich in quality proteins. In the scheme of things, nature has placed the supply of protein so that it is available to nourish the germinating or sprouting plant until the plant can produce its own requirements. Beans are a particularly good source of vegetable proteins. A very large industry has developed through the growing and processing of soybeans, which on a dry-meal basis contain approximately 50% protein. Soybean protein is an important source of protein for human and animal food. Many substitute meat products are produced from soybean protein. Additionally, this protein is used extensively to fortify wheat flour and other foods to improve the nutritional value of such foods.

Of course, a large part of the protein for human food is obtained from animal sources. Products such as meat, milk, eggs, and seafoods serve as sources of a huge quantity of high-quality protein for mankind. The protein from such animal sources originated largely from plants consumed by the animal, but such vegetable proteins have been extensively reconstructed by the chemical processes of the digestive and metabolic systems of the animal. This has resulted in upgrading significantly the quality of such proteins in terms of the requirements for properly nourishing the human system.

In keeping with the phase of our theme which gives recognition to the fact that all material things on our planet are composed of chemical elements, it is proper for us to examine the chemical composition of proteins. In any case, the nature of the chemical composition of all the various nutrients for the human system is of great importance in terms of supplying to such system the exact type of raw material required to make the system function on an optimum basis. It is only on such basis that we may expect a full measure of health and well-being.

The chemical elements contained in all proteins are carbon, oxygen, hydrogen, and nitrogen. Most of the proteins also contain sulfur. These elements are arranged in a systematic pattern to form a chemical molecule known to the chemist as an amino acid. There are 23 of these amino acids in proteins. Each one of the 23 of these compounds is of a different pattern in respect to either the number of atoms of each of the five elements it contains or the order of the arrangement of the elements in the amino acid molecule. Since the proteins are composed of 23 amino acids, we may think of the amino acids as subunits of the proteins or consider them "building blocks" of the proteins.

Each amino acid has a common name and a scientific name. The scientific name describes to the chemist precisely the number of atoms of each element and the location of the atoms of each element in the structural formula of the amino acid molecule. As an example, the common name of one of the amino acids is glycine. The scientific name of glycine is aminoacetic acid. The structural formula for glycine is $H—\overset{\overset{\displaystyle NH_2}{|}}{\underset{\underset{\displaystyle H}{|}}{C}}—COOH$. The symbol N is for the element nitrogen, H for hydrogen, C for carbon, and O for oxygen. The carbon atom having two hydrogen atoms attached to it is known to the chemist as being in the alpha position. If this alpha carbon had a third hydrogen attached to it, instead of the amine group ($—NH_2$), then the structural formula would be that of acetic acid. This illustrates in a relatively simple manner how the chemist readily knows the exact structural formula or precisely the exact number and location of each element in the molecule since the scientific name of glycine (aminoacetic acid) clearly relates it to acetic acid, of which he already knows the structural formula.

Below is a list of the 23 amino acids commonly present in proteins.

Alanine	Leucine
Aspartic Acid	Lysine
Arginine	Methionine
Cysteine	Phenylalanine
Cystine	Proline
Di-iodotyrosine	Serine
Glutamic Acid	Threonine
Glycine	Thyroxine
Histidine	Tryptophan
Hydroxyproline	Tyrosine
Hydroxylysine	Valine
Isoleucine	

Without entering into a complex technical discussion,

one may think of these subunits, the amino acids, as being linked together to form a protein. A protein molecule contains a great number of amino acids linked or bonded together by chemical forces. One of the smaller protein molecules, insulin, contains 51 amino acid units. Another protein, ribonuclease, contains 124 units. The protein in tobacco mosaic virus contains 158. Some proteins contain many hundreds of amino acid units.

Not only the total number of amino acid units, the number of a particular unit, and the ratio of any one unit to any other, but also the sequence of the arrangement of each of the 23 units present in a protein results in forming a different protein, which may have a different function or capability for performing a task. Thus, as an illustration, if a protein has the amino acid glycine adjacent to alanine and the next amino acid in the sequence is serine, then the protein would be different from one which had the serine adjacent to the glycine with the next amino acid in the sequence being alanine. This point may be further illustrated by the rearrangement of letters to spell words. An example would be the word "name," which by a simple rearrangement of the same letters becomes "mane," which is a word with a completely different meaning. Perhaps one can better comprehend the vast number of proteins possible, by the vast number of rearrangements in the sequence of amino acids which theoretically exist, if one thinks of the many words which can be constructed from various combinations of the 26 letters of the English alphabet. The possible combinations of the 23 amino acids in protein molecules is expanded greatly by the fact that in some proteins there are hundreds of amino acids involved, whereas there are no words having nearly that many letters.

Not all proteins are of the same value as nutrients for mankind. The nutrient value or the quality of a protein resides in the number of individual essential amino acids and the quantity of such essential amino acids that are contained in the structure of a given protein. The human and animal body has the ability to synthesize, by the chemical processes constantly operating within it, certain amino acids to make them available to produce the proteins which need to be replaced every minute of a lifetime. But there are some amino acids which are required for the construction of proteins within the body which cannot be synthesized by the chemical processes of the body, and therefore it is essential that these be made available, in the required quantities, as raw materials in the food consumed. This group of 8 amino acids, in the case of the human species, are generally referred to as the essential amino acids. It is the presence of this group of 8 essential amino acids, in ample quantities, which determines the quality of a protein in terms of man.

The accompanying table provides a list of the essential amino acids. Furthermore, it introduces the principle of nitrogen equilibrium, which is simply the relationship between the amount of nitrogen entering the system (through the ingestion of amino acids in proteins) and the excretion of nitrogen as metabolic end products (through feces, urine, and skin), mostly as urea but some as creatinine, uric acid, and small amounts of other nitrogen-bearing compounds. In a healthy adult the intake of nitrogen normally is equal to the output, in which case the system is said to be in nitrogen balance. During illness, fasting, or extensive inadequate protein intake a wastage of tissue occurs; then the output exceeds the intake and a negative balance exists. During the growing period a positive balance needs to be maintained because the body must retain some of the ingested nitrogen (from amino acids in proteins) as newly formed body proteins to build tissue for growth.

QUANTITATIVE REQUIREMENTS OF ESSENTIAL AMINO ACIDS FOR NITROGEN EQUILIBRIUM IN HUMAN ADULTS[1]

	Minimum Grams per Day	
Amino Acids	Male	Female
Isoleucine	0.70	0.45
Leucine	1.10	0.62
Lysine	0.80	0.50
Methionine	0.20 to 1.10[2]	0.35
Phenylalanine	0.30 to 1.10[2]	0.22
Threonine	0.50	0.31
Tryptophan	0.25	0.16
Valine	0.80	0.65

Even though the 8 amino acids listed above are considered to be those which are essential for man to maintain nitrogen equilibrium, arginine and histidine are additionally required for optimal rate of growth of laboratory animals. It is generally assumed that this likewise applies to man.

Nitrogen equilibrium can be established over a wide range of protein intake, from as low as 15 grams to as high as 175 grams per day. This indicates that the quantity of amino acids available to the tissues determines the rate of protein metabolism. There is a continuous and dynamic nitrogen (from amino acids in proteins) metabolism, but the rate is determined by the

---

[1] Adapted from National Academy of Sciences—National Research Council, *Evaluation of Protein Nutrition*, Publication 711.

[2] The amino acid cystine has a sparing effect for methionine, so that when cystine is present the lower amount is required but when absent the higher amount becomes the requirement. The same applies to phenylalanine in the presence or absence of tyrosine, which has a sparing action for phenylalanine.

concentration of the reactants. This is a common principle in virtually all chemical reactions.

If amino acids are required for certain life-sustaining processes, and such amino acids are not available from proteins being ingested, then the human system has the capability to consume some of its own less essential tissue to provide amino acids to carry on the life-sustaining processes. Creating such an amino acid deficiency situation certainly is not in the best interests of the integrity of the body. There may be compelling circumstances, such as in the case of some types of diseases, where one cannot avoid this. But such a situation should never be allowed to occur because of careless nutrition practices. It always needs to be remembered that there is no depot type of storage for proteins as there is for fats.

Another principle of good nutrition which needs to be remembered is that all the essential amino acids must be available at the same time. The proteins in the body are constantly breaking down into their amino acid units to be resynthesized to satisfy the changing requirements of the system. The amino acids derived from proteins in ingested food and from the body proteins form a pool of amino acid raw materials for the system's production of its protein needs. All essential amino acids must be available at the same time. If one of them is absent, even though supplied several hours later, the nutritional effectiveness of the whole group has been reduced. This dramatically illustrates the nutritional inadequacy which can be created by a marginal protein diet. It highlights too the need for having each meal supply the complete number of essential amino acids by way of inclusion of good-quality proteins from several sources. The seafood or steak which you are having for dinner is of no value in upgrading the quality of a low-quality breakfast or lunch. For an optimum level of nutrition each meal must supply a source of the complete list of essential amino acids, and this can be accomplished only by consuming a liberal portion of quality proteins as a part of each meal.

From our discussion it is evident that the biological value of a protein is important. This is determined by the quality of the protein in terms of the essential amino acid content. But it is important to remember that the protein must enter our digestive system in a form in which it is digestible; otherwise the amino acids of which the protein is composed do not become available to the system. In human nutrition this problem largely arises when a protein food, such as a steak, is too well done. Excessive heat denatures the protein, which is another way of saying that the protein has undergone an intramolecular change. Depending on the degree of abuse by excessive exposure to heat, some or most of the protein may have been rendered indigestible and unavailable to the system, and some, or perhaps all, of the vitamins may have been destroyed.

An ample quantity of available protein of high quality in the diet is of great importance. However, it is important too to remember that unless the diet contains a sufficient quantity of carbohydrates and fat to supply calories for energy, and to satisfy certain other chemical needs, the chemical processes will utilize protein for such purposes. It is unlikely that it is nature's intent that protein should preferably follow such a metabolic pathway, but it is a capability of the chemical system of the human organism, which nature has provided, to be certain of a source of energy so long as food of any type is available. It is neither good "biologic economics" nor good monetary economics to fail to supply ample fat or carbohydrates to supply the energy required by the system and thus spare the more precious and more costly protein from having to be used extensively as a source of energy.

The quantity of protein recommended by the Food and Nutrition Board of the National Academy of Sciences-National Research Council (NAS-NRC) is a daily amount of 1 gram per kilogram of body weight on a dry-weight basis of protein. This amounts to 70 grams (2½ ounces) daily for a male weighing 70 kilograms, equal to 154 pounds. This weight of 70 kilograms for a male and 58 (128 pounds) kilograms for a female is used widely in human nutrition as the average "reference man and woman." Thus an average woman would require 58 grams of protein daily or approximately 2 ounces. These amounts anticipate moderate activity in a moderate climate for the period of early adulthood through the remainder of the life span. The foregoing amounts of protein are considered to allow a margin of safety, but there are valid reasons which suggest that a larger amount of protein is desirable.

One cannot be certain at all times of the quality of the protein in the commercially prepared ready-to-eat food products. One does not know to what degree standard food products have been deprived of quality proteins during normal processing, either through elimination of part of the composition or through denaturation by heat or chemicals. Increasing protein intake will increase the sum total of available essential amino acids under such circumstances. Even though a great deal is known about the science of nutrition, we are not in a position to definitely state that an adequate intake constitutes the optimum. As an example, relatively recent scientific data indicates that men after age 50 have a higher requirement for the amino acids lysine and methionine than younger men. Resistance to disease is enhanced by the availability of an ample supply of proteins, since antibody production requires proteins. A high-protein diet appears to be a matter of good common sense to all who are fortunate enough to have it within their reach. As much as 90 grams for the 70-kilogram male and 70 grams for the 58-kilogram female may be more nearly the optimum protein intake than any lower level.

There are clearly defined circumstances for which an

increase in the protein intake is urged. These circumstances are conditions which require the growth of new tissue. In cases of severe injury or surgery new tissue must be generated to repair the damage. In many instances of illness, the chemical processes have consumed some of the proteins of the tissues, due to either fasting or fever, and extra protein intake is indicated to restore nitrogen balance. This highlights the urgent need for a high-quality protein diet in hospitals. In the event the digestive system is unable to tolerate an ample quantity of a high-quality diet which is indicated for the welfare of the body, possibly due to surgery of the digestive system, gastroenteritis, or the like, then intravenous feeding of a protein solution (if indicated, fortified with synthetic amino acids) needs to be employed.

Pregnancy and lactation are circumstances which make it urgent to increase protein intake. Under these circumstances, a woman should certainly increase her protein intake by 20% over the amount considered adequate prior to pregnancy. This assumes that her nutrition was at a satisfactory level for a prolonged period prior to pregnancy. Many young mothers (more than one-third of the births are to women under 21 years) have followed a poor diet consisting too largely of such items as potato chips, candy, soft drinks, and doughnuts. These women are in a very poor state of nutrition to nourish a developing baby and need to increase their protein intake sharply if they are interested in protecting the welfare of their own bodies and properly nourishing their fetuses so that they may deliver normal, healthy babies. A great deal of protein is required to form the multiplicity of types of tissues which are necessary for the development of the complete little body growing daily in the womb. There is no source of this required protein other than the mother's own tissues and the food which she consumes. Likewise, if the baby is breast-fed after birth, the mother will have a heavy output of protein, since human milk is a high-protein product, containing an abundance of essential amino acids. There is no source of these milk proteins other than the mother's own tissues and the food she consumes. There are no circumstances in which protein nutrition becomes a more critical matter than during the period of pregnancy and lactation.

An infant requires a greater amount of protein per unit of body weight than an adult because it needs to continuously produce new tissue for growth in addition to having all the other basic requirements for protein. During the first year of life the increase in body size percentagewise is greater than during any other period. The body weight of a healthy baby will normally double during the first four to five months. The protein requirements during this period are in the range of 2.5 to 3 grams per kilogram (2.2 lb.) body weight, with the requirement gradually declining to about 1.5 to 1.6 grams at the end of the first year of life. The requirement for protein remains at this level for the remainder of the growing period, during the latter part of which it gradually recedes to the level for adulthood.

The consequences of protein deficiency are numerous and may create serious problems. Basically, if there is a dietary protein deficiency, it becomes impossible for the chemical processes to construct the protein molecules which are essential to the normal life processes. In more technical terms, protein synthesis, or anabolism, cannot proceed at the required rate. Thus weight is lost by the adult and growth is retarded in the growing child. The synthesis of hemoglobin is impaired, resulting in anemia. The capacity for forming antibodies may become impaired and consequently the resistance to disease diminished. A prolonged deficiency of protein may cause an accumulation of excessive amounts of fat in the liver due to a deficiency of the methylating amino acid methionine. This in turn may cause degenerative changes resulting in cirrhosis. After full liver function is impaired, direct and indirect stresses of other organs are created, particularly the kidneys and organs of the cardiovascular system. A prolonged protein deficiency may result in a reduced synthesis of plasma proteins which allows the accumulation of an excessive amount of fluid in the intertissue areas. Low protein intake may make it impossible to synthesize such hormones as are of protein composition and thus induce endocrine abnormalities. In advanced cases of protein deficiency, the synthesis of enzymes may be impaired, thereby impairing certain functions of the liver and reducing the content of pepsin for food digestion. An ample supply of protein is indeed a necessity if one wishes to enjoy a full measure of health.

This point of discussion of proteins is probably as appropriate a place as anywhere to introduce the subject of enzymes. The substances known as enzymes are basically protein molecules of a very specific chemical composition in respect to amino acid content. They serve as catalysts of chemical reactions, which is to say that they control chemical reactions, without the molecule of the enzyme being retained as a part of the end product of the reaction catalyzed. The enzymes can use chemical energy available from the food nutrients and can direct it into the necessary pathways to synthesize the chemical compounds required by the system. They are the controlling factor in directing the conversion of chemical energy into mechanical and electrical energy in the body. Enzymes are the controlling factor in determining the particular chemical reactions which constitute the complex series of metabolic processes of the body. They control many essential chemical reactions which thus far have not been carried out outside the body. There are about 700 different enzymes known, each of which directs and controls a specific type of chemical reaction.

The foregoing discussion of proteins may appear to be a lengthy scientific dissertation as part of a book on the subject of health. Nevertheless, it simply skims the surface. Hopefully, the discussion highlights the important basic scientific information which will serve to give the nonspecialist in nutrition the kind of overview which may give a full comprehension of the science behind the guidelines of a sound nutritional program. Hopefully too, this discussion may establish a further comprehension of the fact that a good nutritional program is based on a background of scientific facts and not on someone's pet theory, prejudices, fancy, fantasy, or fad.

In view of the relatively precise scientific guidelines in respect to protein requirements and the many protein-containing foods of a large variation of quality and quantity in protein content, it may look as though the situation necessarily results in a dilemma. But this is not really the case. There are practical solutions available for satisfying human nutritive requirements for protein. The problem can be simplified to one of gaining a bit of basic knowledge regarding the quality and quantity of protein in the common foodstuffs and then consuming liberal quantities of the desirable items. The table of food composition at the end of this book may serve as a useful guide.

As a general principle it is well to keep in mind that protein-bearing products, on a dry-weight basis, derived from animal sources contain the highest percentage content of protein and such protein is of high quality, that is, it contains a substantial amount of the essential amino acids. This necessarily means that meat, milk, eggs, and seafood are the preferred sources of protein. All types of plants contain some protein but in lesser quantity and quality than most of the protein foods from animal sources. Beans, peas, and nuts of all varieties are fairly high in protein of fairly good quality. Soybeans are an outstanding example of a product of plant origin having a high protein content of fairly good quality. The volume of production of soybeans is tremendous (U.S., over 1 billion bushels per year), and the high-protein meal is widely used in animal feeds and for production of high-protein flour, and of pure soybean proteins, for fortifying a variety of food products and for producing simulated meat items. Even though several sources of fairly good-quality plant proteins exist, they do not fully match the quality of most of the proteins from animal sources.

It is evident from the foregoing that the vegetarian theory is not based on reliable scientific information. It must be apparent that the diet of a strict vegetarian is suboptimal from a protein standpoint. If it were not for beans, peas, and nuts in the diet, the strict vegetarian would experience serious difficulties. In areas where such vegetables and animal sources of proteins are not available, as among some tribes in Africa, a very serious and painful protein deficiency disease known as kwashiorkor is prevalent. Of course, there are very few, if any, absolutely strict vegetarians in the advanced countries. Most of the so-called vegetarians obtain some animal proteins by some such routes as milk in their coffee or tea and by eating custards, puddings, pies, cakes, processed recipes, and diet bread, many of which contain protein from an animal source. Even though such source does not supply an adequate amount of essential amino acids, it does undoubtedly serve as a helpful supplement.

Protein quality is often used as a term which is synonymous with biological value. On this basis the protein from eggs is considered to have a biological value of about 100. Wheat has a biological value of 50 with its low content of the important essential amino acid lysine. Theoretically, twice the quantity of wheat protein should be equal in protein value to a given quantity of egg protein, but if the natural wheat product were used, it would concurrently mean the consumption of an excessive amount of starch. On this same biological scale beefsteak has a value of about 90.

This brief illustration indicates the desirability of following a diet which includes food items from several different sources.

As a practical matter many interesting and palatable possibilities exist for a menu which will satisfy the requirements of an optimum level of protein nutrition. A few of these will be explored in the succeeding paragraphs. A bit of knowledge mixed with a bit of ingenuity will suggest many more.

For a breakfast menu the egg has long been and should continue to be a standard item. This supplies about 6 grams of the highest-quality protein. Many people believe that eggs are taboo because of their cholesterol content, but if a satisfactory health program is followed throughout, one need not be concerned about the cholesterol. (A succeeding chapter on cholesterol gives further information on this subject.) There is no valid reason why one should be deprived of the high-quality protein in the egg simply because it contains cholesterol. Eggs too can be prepared in many palatable ways. Thus eggs lend themselves to a variety type of diet on a day-to-day basis. They are good hard-cooked, soft-cooked, poached, scrambled, or scrambled with lox, and as plain omelet, Spanish omelet, ham omelet, cheese omelet, french toast, or Salzburger Nockerlin, and in various other ways. All of the foregoing are familiar to every cook with the possible exception of the Salzburger Nockerlin, which nevertheless is exceptionally delightful. It consists of three egg yolks, three teaspoonsful sugar, three teaspoonsful flour. Beat the egg whites separately and mix the foregoing ingredients. Pour the mix into a hot frying pan which has been greased, preferably with safflower oil. Fry on both sides.

To further increase the protein intake in the breakfast diet a small serving of fish is excellent. The protein content is high and of good quality. It has a high content of many of the B vitamins and trace minerals. If it is an oily fish, it will contain some vitamins A, D, and E and an abundance of polyunsaturated fats. Canned sardines, salmon, and tuna are excellent. Herring preserved in wine sauce or schmaltz herring is very good and practical. Lox is delightful. Mackerel, fresh or salted (with most of the salt leached out), is very acceptable after cooking. Finnan haddie cooked in skim milk is very tasty and a good source of protein and the only one of those named above which contains no oil.

To further increase the protein content of the breakfast diet, one may wish to add a small serving of a high-protein brand cereal or wheat germ meal served with skim milk. Such items add additional amounts of good-quality protein from both the cereal and the milk, as well as B vitamins and vitamin E from wheat germ meal. Wheat germ contains very high-quality protein for a protein from a plant source. The cereal and wheat germ add carbohydrates and the milk adds lactose, so that some of the requirements for nonprotein calories are being satisfied. A slice of bread or toast, with jam if desired (no butter), should be included as a part of the fish and egg course to further add to the nonprotein calorie intake. Fruit juice of choice will make a further contribution.

With the breakfast as suggested in the foregoing paragraphs, a good beginning has been made toward the 70 to 90 grams of required protein for the day. The number of grams such breakfast yields is greatly influenced by the size of portions consumed. But from this type of breakfast it is possible to obtain one-third of the daily requirement. This type of breakfast is certain to provide the full list of essential amino acids and a liberal supply of all the vitamins. But one should remember that breakfast is a very important meal for the protection of the body. It usually is the meal which follows the longest period of time during which no nutrients have been supplied to the system.

After a nutritious breakfast of the foregoing type, the

lunch should be limited unless one is engaged in strenu-
ous physical activity. The lunch should nevertheless be
a balanced type. A glass of milk with a plain dry meat
sandwich with lettuce or a salad of cottage cheese and
fruit or a tuna fish or chicken salad sandwich should do
very well. If an excess of calories is of great concern,
lunch is the most practical time to restrict the intake.

Dinner presents many possibilities to add to the protein intake in a pleasant way. Steaks, prime ribs, roasts,
ham, roast pork, pork chops, lamb, veal, fowl, seafoods
of a wide variety—any of these many comprise the
main course to further add to the protein intake, to
build up to the total requirement for the day. The protein intake at dinnertime may be supplemented by a
soup containing a liberal amount of beans or a salad of
cottage cheese, or a kidney bean salad or a Waldorf
salad with a liberal amount of walnuts. Vegetable items
may be chosen as desired to round out the meal. If
noodles, spaghetti, or similar items are served instead
of potatoes, the protein intake may be increased somewhat because some brands of these items have high-
protein soy flour added to enhance their nutritional
value. Lima or other bean items or peas can further
add protein of fairly good quality to the meal. If a soup
is served, a vegetable soup containing a liberal quantity
of beans or fish chowder can make a worthwhile contribution of protein. Ice milk as dessert, instead of ice
cream or any one of the many high-calorie dessert
items, can make this course pleasant and yet contribute
a significant amount of protein.

If for special reasons a large lunch was consumed,
dinner might consist of some simple high-protein dish
such as fish chowder. For those who enjoy engaging in
and eating home cooking, a very nourishing fish chowder can easily be made which is of high nutritional
value, relatively low in calories, and virtually a complete meal. Simply heat skim milk nearly to the boiling
point and add fish cut into large bite-size pieces to-

gether with cut-up celery, potatoes, and onions. Season with Worcestershire sauce, a hot pepper finely cut or Tabasco, and some black pepper, each item in quantities to suit one's taste. Monosodium glutamate may be added to enhance the flavor, if desired, but for anyone on a salt-free diet it should be omitted. (Pay no attention to the unfavorable publicity monosodium glutamate has received in the public press, for it is the sodium salt of glutamic acid, one of the amino acids of proteins, and is completely harmless in the recommended quantities.) Slowly cook the foregoing mixture so that it boils slowly for about one-half hour. No butter is required. A small amount of salt may be used, but this is not necessary to make it palatable. If fish from salt water is used, a small amount of salt is present from that source. Usually nonoil fish, such as cod, hake, or haddock is used, but fish of a medium level of oil content, such as ocean perch, flounder, or mackerel, is acceptable. The nonoily fish helps to keep the calories low, but the oily types add some valuable polyunsaturated fat to the diet. When this dish is properly seasoned, it is delicious and contains an abundance of high-quality protein from the fish and milk. If skim milk is used, and no butter, it is relatively low in calories. In addition to the protein, it supplies milk sugar from the milk and starch from the potatoes, celery, and onions which virtually make it a high-quality balanced meal. A supply for several days may be made, as it keeps well under normal refrigeration.

It may be well to note that excellent high-quality protein diets may be prepared most economically from fish and poultry. The protein quality from both of these sources is very high and the fat content is lower than in beef where there is marbling. Much of the pork and beef is high in saturated fats. Thus a lower-calorie diet can be followed by the use of fish, broilers, and turkeys if these are extensively used as the major source of protein. Whatever fat is ingested from fish or poultry is largely unsaturated, whereas the fat in red meat is mostly saturated. If the skin of fish or poultry is removed, the fat from these sources is much lower in cholesterol than the fat from red meats. Of course, everyone likes to enjoy a good steak, prime ribs, a fine roast of beef or pork, ham, lamb, or pork chops once in a while, but the above scientific guidelines are worth keeping in mind.

There are many types of diets, such as for infants, for pregnant women, and for those with various types of chronic ailments, in which abnormal circumstances must be considered in the nutrition program. In many of such situations virtually a "tailor-made" diet has to be designed which does not place a burden on the system, yet fulfills the nutritional needs as best one can. The personal physician will need to design such diets to fit the individual circumstances. Nevertheless, the same scientific facts regarding nutrition do apply, but these have to be coordinated with the knowledge of the limitations placed on the nutritional program by the malfunction in the system which creates the special situation.

It is not advocated that only protein foods be consumed. The examples cited are merely illustrations of how one can design a program of good protein nutrition to fulfill the requirements of the optimum protein intake for the general population. By checking the types and quantities of food consumed against the tables in the Appendix, one can readily calculate approximately how closely the protein intake matches the desired optimum. It should always be remembered that even though an ample quantity of all nutrients is very important, having ample protein is of the most critical importance. This is so because such a large percentage of the tissues of the body consist of protein. So many of the life-sustaining chemical processes require a large quantity and variety of proteins. Protein has the versatility of serving as a nutrient for a source of energy, in addition to performing these other functions.

These discussions of the chemistry of the proteins hopefully will serve to establish in the mind of the reader the concept that solid science underlies a good nutritional program. The discussions hopefully too will give the reader helpful guidelines for improving the personal nutritional program and thereby serve as an aid to more healthful living.

FOUR

MINERALS:
THE MINE WITHIN YOU

by

**RUTH CAREY, IRMA VYHMEISTER &
JENNIE HUDSON**

—Common Sense Nutrition

"EAT your spinach, Son. It has minerals in it." Mothers throughout much of the world coax their children to eat with similar statements.

"What's *minerals?*" the child may ask.

"Minerals are . . . well . . . something for your blood. I don't know. Anyway they are good for you." And with that, most mothers feel relieved to let the subject drop.

Of course, the mothers are right. Spinach does contain minerals. And so do bananas, bread, eggs, milk, beans, and most foods. And minerals *are* "good for you." They are essential elements in the blood—and in the nerves, muscles, and other tissues. They build bones and teeth. Other functions are coming to be understood, but much still remains to be learned about minerals. One thing is certain: they are essential.

If you could extract all of the minerals from your body, you would have a heap weighing about six and a half pounds. It would consist mostly of calcium and phosphorus, with some magnesium, sodium, potassium, iron, iodine, and about twenty other minerals, some in such minute amounts that they are called "trace elements."

The minerals found in the body are sometimes grouped as macrominerals (calcium, phosphorus, magnesium, potassium, sodium, chlorine, sulfur) and microminerals (iron, manganese, copper, and iodine). In addition some of the trace elements are known to be essential for body functions (cobalt, fluorine, zinc, selenium, molybdenum), some appear to be essential (chromium), but the functions of some are not known (aluminum, arsenic, boron, bromine, cadmium, lead, nickel, silicon, strontium, vanadium).

Calcium makes up about half of the body's six and one half pounds of minerals, and phosphorus about one-fourth. The remaining macrominerals together account for another pound and a half. The microminerals, mostly iron, weigh little more than one-tenth of an ounce.

The bones and teeth contain the bulk of the body's minerals, but minerals are essential in other parts of the body too. Thyroxin contains iodine, vitamin B_{12} contains cobalt, hemoglobin has iron, and so on.

Calcium and Phosphorus. The skeleton, the framework to which muscles are attached making movement possible, is composed principally of three minerals: calcium, phosphorus, and magnesium. Teeth are built of the same materials.

The teeth and bones contain 99 percent of the calcium and 70 to 80 percent of the phosphorus in the body, so these minerals are sometimes classed together. The National Research Council recommends the same allowances for both except during the first year of life.

Calcium and phosphorus are not the only nutrients essential to bones and teeth, however. Magnesium, fluorine, manganese, vitamins A, C, and D, and even protein are all in some way involved.

Calcium is also needed for muscles, nerves, blood clotting, and some enzyme activity. Yet calcium is a most frequently lacking nutrient in United States diets. No wonder adults, as well as children, are encouraged to drink milk, since it has a high content of calcium easily utilized by the body. One cup of milk furnishes about 280 miligrams of calcium. Two cups a day with an otherwise adequate diet, should provide for adult needs.

Other foods which are good to fair sources of calcium are milk products, greens (including collards, dandelion, kale, mustard, and turnips), other vegetables, some fruits and nuts, and most of the legumes.

You may have heard that some foods are "calcium robbers." It is true that chard, beet greens, spinach, and rhubarb contain oxalic acid which forms an insoluble salt with calcium, but these foods are not usually eaten in great quantities. And they are believed not to affect the calcium utilization of other foods eaten at the same meal; therefore they are really not important in connection with calcium. Something important to note however, is that rhubarb leaves contain high concentrations of oxalic acid and some other deleterious substances. They should never be eaten, since they are not safe, even in small amounts.

Whole wheat and other whole grain cereals contain phytic acid which binds calcium so that it apparently is not absorbed. However, Drs. Wohl and Goodhart* point out that the body must be able under some circumstances to adapt to high intakes of phytic acid since whole tribes have lived in apparent health using enough whole wheat theoretically to cause a loss of more calcium than consumed.

Phosphorus might be described as one of the busiest minerals. It is an essential factor in the metabolism of carbohydrates, fats, and proteins, is part of the buffer system that maintains the body's acid-base balance, is in the cytoplasm of all cells, and is a part of the genes that transmit hereditary characteristics. All this and more is in addition to its functions in the bones and teeth.

The diet will probably have sufficient phosphorus if calcium and protein needs are met. The recommended allowance for phosphorus is the same as for calcium, 800 miligrams a day for adults with additional amounts during pregnancy and lactation, and with varying allowances for children depending upon age.

Among the good food sources of phosphorus are milk and milk products; dried beans, peas, and other legumes; nuts, especially peanuts and brazil nuts; oatmeal and other whole grain cereals; eggs; meats; fish; and fowl.

---

*Michael G. Wohl and Robert S. Goodhart, *Modern Nutrition in Health and Disease*, fourth edition, Lea and Febiger, 1968.

Vitamin D, formed in the skin by the action of sunshine, is essential for the absorption of calcium and phosphorus. Normally the calcium in the body is maintained in balance between the bony tissues and fluids by two hormones, parathormone and calcitonin, aided by vitamin D.

Without sufficient vitamin D, calcium, and phosphorus, a child may develop the soft, bowed bones of rickets, a condition frequently observed in places with little sunshine. In these areas children may be given vitamin D preparations, cod or other fish liver oils. An adult form of rickets, osteomalacia, was common in purdah women in India and Mohammendan lands who were confined indoors without benefit of sunlight.

Magnesium. Your body normally contains about an ounce of magnesium, which cooperates with calcium and phosphorus to form bones and teeth. Magnesium is also important to the heart, nerves, and muscles.

Alcoholics may have low levels of magnesium, but normal people seldom suffer from magnesium deficiency since it is widely available in foods. The National Research Council recommends a magnesium allowance of 300-400 milligrams daily for adults, increased to 450 milligrams during pregnancy and lactation, and amounts varying with age in infancy and childhood.

Magnesium is found in largest quantity in nuts, whole grains, beans, peas, soybeans, and in green leafy vegetables since it is part of the structure of chlorophyll.

Iron. The three grams of iron in your body would be enough to make only a small nail, but this mininutrient does maximum work.

The liver and spleen store approximately one gram of iron. The rest is in the hemoglobin, in the myoglobin of muscles, and in various enzymes.

Throughout life the body continually needs iron, although it uses and reuses every bit it gets. Children and teen-agers need comparatively more iron than adults.

Women during pregnancy and lactation, in fact through the child-bearing years, have a high requirement. Their recommended allowance (18 milligrams a day) is nearly twice the 10 milligrams recommended for men.

Sufficient iron to meet the recommended allowances for women is frequently not included in the average diet. However, by taking care to choose foods rich in iron daily, a woman can avoid anemia due to iron deficiency.

Among the good iron sources are egg yolk, whole wheat, nuts, dates, dried fruits, beans, lentils, green leafy vegetables, oatmeal, liver, molasses, and meats.

Iodine. Not many years ago iodine deficiency became recognized as a public health problem. Simple goiter, which is an enlargement of the thyroid gland in the neck, was common; and it was found to be caused by lack of sufficient iodine in the food. Goiter was observed especially among people who lived far from the sea, as in the Great Lakes region in the United States, the Alpine mountains in Europe, or the Andean plateaus of South America.

With the addition of a small amount of iodine to table salt, simple goiter can be largely eradicated. Those living near the sea, eating sea foods, or those using iodized salt get enough iodine to meet the recommended daily allowances of 80 to 140 micrograms for adults. The allowances for children vary with age and sex.

Fluorine. Recently it has been discovered that adequate fluorine helps to maintain strong bones and to prevent dental caries (cavities). It appears that it may be beneficial in osteoporosis, a demineralization of the bones, usually observed in older persons.

Since dental caries are rampant in the United States, fluoridation of water has been suggested and is a subject of considerable controversy.

The addition of fluorine to water of low fluorine content has appeared to result in fewer dental caries. The amount that will protect teeth from caries is one to one and a half parts of fluorine per million parts of water. In concentrations higher than 1.5 parts per million, mottling of the teeth may result. Where water has excessive fluorine as in the Texas Panhandle and in certain regions of Colorado, mottling of the teeth is quite common among residents.

Copper. Copper helps to form hemoglobin although it is not a part of it. Copper is found in certain enzymes and ceruloplasmin, a protein in the blood.

If the diet is adequate in other respects, it should provide sufficient copper.

Cobalt. Cobalt is a part of vitamin B_{12}, and its function is linked to that of the vitamin.

Cattle and other ruminants can form their own vitamin B_{12} if their feed contains sufficient cobalt. If pastures lack cobalt, these animals become anemic and have other symptoms that can be cured by adding either vitamin B_{12} or cobalt to the feed.

Humans cannot synthesize vitamin B_{12} in their tissues, so they must take it in their food. Since cobalt is at the core of vitamin B_{12}, sufficient vitamin B_{12} in the diet assures sufficient cobalt. Vitamin B_{12} has been called the "animal protein factor" because it is found almost exclusively in animal foods. Vegetable foods either do not have any or have very negligible amounts.

Zinc. Only minute quantities of zinc are found in the body, but it has important functions. Its highest concentrations are in the bones, skin, liver, and blood. It is involved in a number of enzyme systems and has been found to promote wound healing. Authorities in Iran and Egypt have reported an anemia accompanied by dwarfism and attributed to zinc deficiency.

The usual dietary includes ten to fifteen milligrams of zinc. Zinc can be toxic and cause poisoning if taken in too large amounts. It is widely distributed in foods, so there is ordinarily little chance of lack in the diet. Best sources are wheat germ, yeast, liver, and sea foods.

Sodium, Potasium, and Chlorine. These minerals help to maintain the acid-base balance and have other essential functions. They are in adequate supply in the average diet.

Selenium, Manganese, Molybdenum. Selenium, known as "factor 3," is associated with vitamin E functions. Animals of some species have been found to require selenium, but too much can be toxic. "Blind staggers" is due to selenium poisoning and may occur when animals graze on alkali pastures.

Manganese and molybdenum assist certain enzymes at their work.

Acid-base Balance. If a person comes to your door selling "alkalizing" concoctions, watch out. What you buy may be more harmful than helpful. You may have heard that there are acid-forming foods and alkaline-forming foods. You may have been told that you must beware of acid-forming foods, and so perhaps you feel somewhat apprehensive.

Actually the body has ways in which to maintain the delicate balance between the acids and bases formed in the utilization of foods. When you burn wood in your fireplace, ashes are left. When food is eaten, we speak of its being burned in the body and forming an ash or residue.

For instance if you were to burn cereals, cheese, eggs, meats, fish, poultry, walnuts, peanuts, filberts, Brazil nuts, lentils, macaroni, and noodles in the laboratory, they would leave an ash residue. On analysis the ash would be found to have an excess of phosphorus, sulfur, and chlorine. They are components of an acid ash, therefore these foods are said to leave acid residues.

On the other hand if vegetables, potatoes, fruits, milk, molasses, legumes, and some nuts were burned, these ashes would contain an excess of calcium, potassium, sodium, and magnesium. These foods, and others that may have an acid taste, leave an alkaline or base ash.

Here is the way in which the body acts when confronted with an excess of either acid or alkaline residue. The body contains substances called buffers which can combine with either acids or bases. If excess acid is formed, buffers neutralize it. If the excess is base, buffers neutralize it also.

If the body has too much acid, the kidneys will normally make the urine more acid and thus eliminate the excess. The same is true with an excess base. The buffers, the kidneys, and the lungs will, under normal conditions, neutralize the acids and bases. In this way the blood and other fluids are maintained in a slightly alkaline state.

A food's being an acid- or alkaline-ash yielder has nothing to do with its taste. For instance, orange juice tastes acid because of the organic acids in it. But these acids usually combine with basic substances leaving an alkaline ash in the body. Cereals and meat, which do not taste acid, render acid ash.

A normally healthy person who eats an adequate diet with a variety of fruits and vegetables, milk products, cereals, and protein foods, does not need to concern himself about the body's acid-base balance. It works automatically.

Water

When Sir Edmund Hillary and his expedition first reached the summit of Mount Everest in 1953, it was said that an adequate water supply was the greatest factor in their success. Other expeditions before theirs had not made proper provision for water to balance the losses, and the climbers had to return, their goal not reached.

"The sea within us," as one author puts it, accounts for more than half the body weight of an adult person.

We may go without food for weeks, but we can go only a few days without water. It has been suggested by nutrition scientists that a person may lose all his glycogen, all his fat, and half his protein without real danger, but losing just 10 percent of his body water is serious, and 20 to 22 percent is fatal.

Water may escape from the body through the lungs, the kidneys, the skin, and the gastrointestinal tract. These losses must be constantly replenished.

Why is water so important? Simply because it has so many jobs to do. Water is part of every cell. It transports all the foodstuffs to the cells, and the operations within the cells occur in a watery medium. Substances in the body have to be maintained in solution, and secretions and wastes must be carried out of the cells by water. Water regulates the body temperature, adjusting to the water losses and the changes in the surroundings. Four quarts of water are constantly circulating in the body as part of the blood.

Children lose water easily since their bodies contain proportionately more water than adults, and they have comparatively larger surface areas and higher metabolic rates. Thus an infant or a child has to drink water more often. Dehydration may occur very quickly if a child vomits or has diarrhea or is exposed to too much heat.

In hot weather or while driving through the desert be sure to have plenty of water to drink. If you do hard work in hot surroundings, not only water but also salt should be replenished if the loss is persistent.

Six to eight glasses of fluid a day is recommended. When you get up in the morning try drinking a glass or more of fresh water. It will perk you up and start your day well.

FIVE

ANSWERS TO YOUR QUESTIONS ABOUT HEALTH

by

MAX WARMBRAND

—*Health Today* magazine

What is the difference between natural and synthetic vitamins?

Natural vitamins are living, vital substances which are part of the whole food grown in nature. Synthetic vitamins are chemicals produced out of coal-tar products. Natural vitamins are more beneficial than synthetic because they also contain allied nutrients of great importance to us.

What is Carob?

Also known as "St. John's Bread," carob is the fruit of an evergreen tree found principally in the Mediterranean area. It tastes exactly like chocolate, but unlike chocolate, it is very rich nutritionally, containing vitamins, minerals, natural sugar and proteins. It can be used in any of the ways that chocolate is used.

What is the definition of organic food?

Organic food is food grown in soil which has not been subjected to chemical treatment of any kind but fed by compost and natural mulch. The plants themselves are never chemically sprayed for protection against insects or grubs, or stimulated chemically for production or growth.

Is is true that one deficiency in nutrients can throw the total nutritional balance off?

It is true that one deficiency in *essential* nutrients can unbalance the process of nutritional synthesis. There are at least 40 nutrients which cannot be made in the body, and are essential to good health. They include: amino acids, vitamins, minerals and a fatty acid. They all work in harmony, and a deficiency in one could upset the production of about 10,000 different compounds. The point is that many essential nutrients are lost in refining and processing foods. This is why it is necessary to eat *un*refined, *un*processed foods to maintain good health. Since this may be difficult to do entirely and consistently, it is a good policy to use supplements of vitamins, minerals and proteins in their natural form; as well as fruits and vegetables, wherever possible, as Nature gives them to us.

What is the meaning of poly-unsaturated?

Poly-unsaturated describes a fatty acid particle with certain hydrogen atoms missing. There are 3 fatty acids known as essential: linoleic, linolenic and arachidonic. They are all found in vegetable oils and are necessary to the utilization of cholesterol and *saturated* fats which are solid animal fats. Soy, sunflower, safflower and peanut oils are good sources of essential fatty acids.

Please explain essential amino acids.

Essential amino acids are the amino acids the body requires for growth and rebuilding. As links in the protein chain, amino acids are necessary to human metabolism. There are about 30 of them; the body manufactures about 22 and the rest must be found in the food we eat. We should make sure we get our amino acids from natural sources, such as soft-blend cheese, lean fish or fowl, or any lean meat in small amounts. Also nuts and natural brown rice.

Are food additives invariably harmful?

Natural, unprocessed food, free of chemicals (more than 3,000 different chemicals are being added to processed food in America these days) has to provide more nutritional benefit than food of uncertain value. This is the most generous way of putting it. Some additives have been proved harmful and are still being used; others have never been tested; still others combine or are stored in harmful degrees and amounts. When we take care of our soil and stop abusing it with artificial fertilizers and chemicals—the soil will give us all the food we need; the kind of food that can protect itself against pests.

What is the best way to eliminate the chemicals from our drinking water?

Most chemicals—but not the valuable minerals—will disappear with boiling the water for 10 minutes or so. Or, let the water stand in an open container overnight.

What are the important minerals to include in the diet?

Calcium, copper, iodine, iron, magnesium, potassium and sulphur are all essential minerals. One of the richest single sources of minerals is seaweed, which can be obtained at health food stores as powdered kelp or in conjunction with other powdered vegetables as a general seasoning.

SIX

HONEY, THE REJUVENATOR

by

VIRGINIA CASTLETON THOMAS

—My Secrets of Natural Beauty

HONEY as a food was recognized as a life-sustainer even in pre-Biblical days. Cavemen learned to grab combs of honey from hidden hives, as they warded off the stings of a million angry bees, because of the life-giving and delicious properties of this amber nectar. Honey has been used both as a food and as a cosmetic throughout the centuries. As a source of quick energy because of its predigested natural sugars, honey has no equal. Easily assimilated, its vitamins and minerals boost its value as a health-giving food.

Those same vitamins and minerals turn it into a powerhouse cosmetic when a poorly nourished body produces a skin that is clogged and muddy. Repeated applications of tissue-building honey will bring a glow of color where none existed before.

In addition, honey's bacteria-destroying actions aid patches of inflamed skin. The soothing, thick liquid that heals and nourishes is one of the finest of all skin foods.

Balms, lotions and unguents using honey as a main ingredient have been found to repair sensitive skins that cannot tolerate much activity. Roughened hands dipped into vats of honey in primitive fashion lose their coarsened texture. Bit by bit the healing and beautifying properties of this wonder food were discovered and praised and put to good use.

Today we know the hygroscopic nature of honey attracts and holds moisture to the skin, thus restoring dried, aging tissue at least as long as the applications of honey are used.

Of such great value is the bee industry that all parts of honey production can be used. Beeswax itself is the basis of all good lipsticks, and if one has the proper molds, it is possible to produce a lipstick without the coal tar dyes that keep the lips of women around the world in a continual state of peeling.

Not only the wax, but pollen, carried on the tiny legs of the bees as they dip in and out of blossoms in search of sweet nectar to convert to honey, enriches the honey itself. Pollen has been called nature's richest food. It is small wonder that nutritional richness such as this brings so many beautifying and healing qualities with its use.

Of course, as with any sugar, too much honey as a food should not be consumed. For all its healthy qualities, because of its sugar conent, it should be taken in moderation (and sometimes not at all—particularly by diabetics or hypoglycemics). But there is no limit to its external application, for although only a fraction is absorbed by the skin, it is enough to produce the effects we are after.

Honey can restore a more youthful appearance by the simplest dab on the face or in complicated creams and lotions. Here is a trial facial: splash warm water across a freshly washed face. Do not use any of the other applications suggested in this book, other than perhaps an astringent lotion after cleansing. Otherwise, you place a film barrier over the very pores you are trying to reach. Reserve your creams for later.

Having moistened your face, dip two fingers into a teaspoon of raw, unheated honey. In upward sweeping motions, lightly spread it into every area of your face. Be sure your hair is drawn back and your face fully exposed to the edges of the ear lobes and the top of the forehead for this facial honey bath.

Allow the honey to remain for twenty minutes before rinsing away with warm water. Daily applications of honey can refine and soften skin that has hardened from exposure of poor care. Honey is also helpful to use after removing makeup. Directly after its use, a final rinse in a mixed solution of apple cider vinegar and water will bring a further glow to the skin.

There are always means at hand to combat early wrinkles. And the glory of using one's kitchen as a beauty laboratory is that many of the needed ingredients are already there. As long as you keep a jar of raw, unheated honey on your shelf, half the battle against incipient wrinkles is won.

One quick and remedial recipe combines one teaspoon of honey with two tablespoons of sweet cream. Before milk was homogenized, you could simply lift the cream from the top of the bottle of milk. But if you don't have access to fresh, certified, raw milk, you will have to resort to buying either light cream, sometimes called coffee cream, or heavy whipping cream. Be sure that it is not a milk "food" or other substitute.

Beat the ingredients together and apply to a freshly scrubbed, rinsed and dried face. With the fingertips, pat the mixture into creases and lines.

With a gentle rubbing action, saturate the grooved lines, and as you apply the honey and cream, spread the lines on the face apart. Do not pull or work roughly. Smooth the area instead, and attempt to uncrease the lines.

This is a quickie treatment that can soften the early wrinkling areas around the eyes, mouth and on the forehead. The practice could beneficially become a morning ritual, accompanying breakfast preparation and rinsed away afterward.

Another kitchen treatment using honey with minimum preparation is to mix one-half teaspoon of apple cider vinegar or lemon juice with two tablespoons of honey. Blend together and spread over the face. Allow this to remain on for fifteen or twenty minutes before rinsing away in warm water and blotting the skin dry. This softens and deep cleans, leaving the skin refreshed and free of accumulated oils that a cleansing cream cannot reach.

These mixtures are also excellent for the neck. In fact, this part of the body is usually in as much need of attention as the face and often neglected. One's glance simply doesn't begin and end with the face, but continues over the full expanse of both face and neck.

Honey and almonds in combination is one of the finest cosmetic teams we have. The qualities of both have long been recognized by women around the world who have mastered the art of looking their best at all times. In earlier days there was an excellent commercial preparation using the two items alone.

But more glamorous products seem to have pushed aside this simple, effective skin preserver and rejuvenator. So here is the old recipe, in all its grand simplicity. It is really like having a pot of gold on hand to have this delightful potion on your cosmetic shelf.

Buy a one-pound jar of U.S.P. lanolin (which means it is approved for pharmaceutical use). Choose the hydrous kind which does not require mixing with water. You will need one-half pound of the lanolin in the following recipe; save the remainder for other recipes.

Place one-fourth pound of raw honey in the top of a double boiler, and as it warms, beat in one-half pound of lanolin. As this melts, add one-half cup of sweet almond oil and stir until well blended.

Remove from the heat and beat thoroughly with an electric or hand beater. Get a complete emulsification and then pour into convenient-size jars. Keep all but the jar you are using in the refrigerator. Label the jars carefully so they aren't mistaken for food.

Use the cream liberally over neck, face and elbows. It still has all the magic it had when our grandmothers stepped out smelling of honey and almond cream.

Honey water as a rinse is handed down to us in various recipes. Since it has been in recorded use from the heyday of the Roman empire, there has been ample time to experiment and improve it. Nevertheless, it remains much like the original.

HONEY WATER

4 ounces honey	¼ ounce cloves
½ ounce grated lemon peel	½ ounce nutmeg
½ ounce grated orange peel	2 ounces rose water
½ ounce benzoin	2 ounces elder flower water
½ ounce storax	12 ounces ethyl alcohol

Pour the honey into a two-quart glass jar and add the lemon and orange peel, benzoin, storax, cloves and nutmeg. Stir together to blend. Add the remaining ingredients and beat together. Place a lid on the jar and shake together thoroughly. Allow the mixture to steep for three days, shaking frequently, and then filter and bottle.

This fragrant water was used daily in Roman households and comes to us through the centuries as a mixture of great merit.

Honey comes to the rescue again, after a summer's sun produces blotches of brown and red on the throat and neck. When mixed with oatmeal, it brings about a softening and clearing, since the oatmeal serves as a mild bleach. The following combination, if used nightly and rinsed away each morning, will eventually eliminate the speckled appearance that is so aging.

Mix the following items together until you have an easily spreadable paste: One ounce of honey, one teaspoon of lemon juice, two unbeaten egg whites, one-half teaspoon sweet almond oil and enough oatmeal powder to make a smooth paste. Try whirling a handful of old-fashioned oatmeal in the blender for this. Or reduce oatmeal to a powder in a nut grinder. Have the mixture moist, but not dripping when you apply it to your throat and neck.

SEVEN

RELAXING YOUR WAY TO YOUTHFUL HEALTH

by

CARLSON WADE

—Health Today magazine

RECENTLY, I was called for an interview on a radio show on which a noted performer was the guest star. He was his usual relaxed self right up to air time. The rest of us, however, all felt the mounting tension as we waited for the producer to give the signal that we were on the air.

The producer raised his arm for the signal. Then with only ten seconds to go, this famed performer dropped the script. Panic broke loose—in everyone but this star performer. While actors, agency men, stage hands, and musicians scrambled to pick up the fluttering pages of the script, the performer nonchalantly bent down, picked up the elusive first page, winked at me, then came in exactly on cue. That night he gave a tremendous performance without any fuss whatsoever! His absolutely relaxed attitude made me feel so calm that I went through my interview with the same casual, contented and self-confident manner.

If there is to be any "secret" of relaxation, it is the ability to remain calm when others feel harassed and confused. It is the ability to feel secure and safe regardless of pressures. With surprisingly simple mental and physical exercises, you can develop your ability to relax your way to better health.

RELAXATION BEGINS WITH CALM NERVES. It is said that 7 out of 10 of the people who file into doctors' offices with palpitations, extraneous and light beats of the heart, speeding pulse, or indigestion are told by their physicians, "It's your nerves. You must learn how to relax." Nerves are part of the chain reaction the emotions cause through the physical mechanisms of the nervous system and the internal glands. In turn, they are part of the chain reaction with which the balanced chemistry of our bodies affects our relaxation-power.

You have three basic nerve systems that influence your ability to relax and your ability to meet tensions with natural inner tranquility:

Central Nerve System. Controlled by your conscious,

this "central" or "voluntary" system is one that tells you to eat when hungry, to cover yourself up when cold, to laugh when you feel like it.

Peripheral Nerve System. This deals solely with your sense organs connected with seeing, hearing, smelling, feeling and tasting.

Autonomic Nerve System. This is involved completely with internal activity and it controls the so-called smooth muscles (those of the internal organs, arteries, veins) with its branches reaching into every body cell and tissue. It controls your heartbeat, your breathing, the expansion and contraction of blood vessels, as well as the process of food digestion, storage and release for body use. Your conscious will cannot command the autonomic nervous system. *Your emotions influence this system.* Become tense, fearful, worried, nervous, upset, angry, on edge, and your autonomic system reacts to influence your heart, respiration, arterial system and the digestion of food.

Millions of neurons (collections of nerve cells) make up a nerve fiber. These nerves are as much an actual physical part of your body as your tongue or bladder. Like telephone wires, these nerves run throughout every part of your body, performing every function, both mental and physical, voluntary and involuntary.

Yes, your nerve cells possess temperaments of irritability, adaptability and conductivity just as a human personality. You must keep these tiny but hair-trigger delicate live wire nerves in good emotional condition to be able to relax your way to better health.

MAKE RELAXATION A PART OF LIFE. "If you should individually achieve calmness and harmony in your own person, you may depend upon it that a wave of imitation will spread from you as surely as the circles spread outward when a stone is dropped into a lake." So advised noted professor-writer William James (1842-1910) on building relaxation into your way of life.

It is true, of course, that a half century or so ago,

America was still, in large part, the land of the shade-speckled village and the old mill stream. Life, though earnest, was relatively uncomplicated. There was no wild frenzy to crowd 60 frantic minutes into every frantic hour. There were fewer places to go and people were not in a hurry to get there. Walking was a *natural* means of mobility rather than a prescribed form of exercise.

What has happened over the years need not be written here. Suffice it to say that we have cranked, geared, whirled and wheeled the world we live in to a pulse-pounding, breath-taking pace. Day after day, the alarm clock sends us off and running.

Unfortunately, while we have entered an age of new-fashioned marvel and momentum, we have done so with the same old-fashioned bodies. In our struggle to keep step with our inventions, we have let ourselves run ragged. The "body machine" is neglected in favor of the mechanical machine. The "body machine" runs down but the mechanical machine gets its regular treatments and cares. No one is suggesting we go back to the horse-and-buggy days but it would be wise if we could go back to that same feeling of relaxation that characterized those pastoral farm and city folk. *It can be done!*

WHAT IS RELAXATION? The word "relax" is taken from the Latin *re* meaning "again" and *laxus* meaning "loose." Basically, it calls for loosening up the taut nerves and emotions and become pleasurably flaccid. In the words of the Roman lyric poet, Catullus (87 B.C.–45 B.C.): "Ahhh, what is more blessed than to put care aside, when the mind lays down its burden, and spent with distant travel, we come home again and rest on the couch we longed for?"

In today's hustle and bustle of modern civilization, in the frenzied pace of newer and newer discoveries, in the urge to get more and more of whatever there is to get, so few of us rest. Relaxation may be thought of as a lost art. Yet, even in this "Age of Anxiety" it is pos-

sible to relax by means of some few exercises and an
emotional understanding, as well. After all, just as tension can make you sick—*relaxation can make you well!*

Relaxation is a required study at Barnard College.
The officials consider relaxation so important that their
gym courses often end up with 10-minute relaxing ses-
sions.

Especially tense girls are encouraged to attend
"relaxation" twice a week. Every student gets a chart
with relaxing exercises to practice alone, as well as
being taught to recognize such symptoms of tension as
nail-chewing, lip-biting, insomnia, eye-batting, stutter-
ing, garbled words, garbled thoughts, headache.

SIMPLE EXERCISE. Professor Marion Streng teaches
the girls to wilt like daisies in easy steps—first, letting
the arms droop, then their heads, followed by relaxation of their upper torsos until their bodies fall to a
sitting position. From this sitting position, the girls can
easily flop down to complete rest. Try this tonight when
you are ready for sleep.

Another way to relax is to locate the tension in your
muscles and correct it. Consciously tense that particular
muscle—the frown wrinkles in your forehead, for example—then let go. It is with your jaw that you grit
teeth in rage, or clench them in determination.

RELAX YOUR HANDS. Tense your hands, then let
them go. Frequently, typists and those who use their
hands, find that shaking the hands from the wrists in a
dangling fashion relieves their hand and wrist tension.

RELAX YOUR TUMMY. Are you living as if you were
expecting a blow in the belly—with your subconscious
making your abdominal muscles constantly on the defensive? With this is the vicious circle of the brain re-
ceiving defensive messages from the abdominal muscles
and the worried brain tensing them. Breathe deeply
from your belly. As the diaphragm smoothly contracts
and lets go, this gentle massage is applied to the entire
abdominal area.

INSTANT RELAXATION. When your bus or train is annoyingly delayed, breathe in very deeply. Draw your abdomen in and up against your spinal column as much as possible. Hold your stomach close to your back for the count of ten—then release your breath. Do this a few times and you will start yawning. *When you relax your jaw and mouth, you are half-relaxed already!* Yawning is a fine way to create a feeling of euphoria of mind and body!

In *How to Relax In A Busy World,* Floyd and Eve Corbin tell us, "If you have been in the habit of inviting negative thoughts—jealousy, envy, resentment and self-pity, think of these as intruders in your mind. The old Chinese saying fits here: 'You cannot stop the birds of the air from flying over your head, but you need not let them nest in your hair!'

"Face and define your troubles. Gather knowledge about them from every good source. Confide your worries to God. Do all you can about the situation that is causing them. Don't contaminate your friends and loved ones with them."

7 MIND-RELAXING STEPS
TO BETTER HEALTH

Famed surgeon, Maxwell Maltz, M.D., author of *Psycho-Cybernetics,* offers these gems of advice on how to ease tensions and help yourself relax your way to better health:

1. *Get The Happiness Habit.* Smile inside, and make this feeling a part of you. Create a happy world for yourself; look forward to each day. Even if some shadows blot out the sunshine, there is always something to feel good about.

2. *Declare War on Negative Feelings.* Don't let unrealistic worries eat away at you! When negative thoughts invade your mind, fight them. Ask yourself why you, who have every natural right to be happy, must spend your waking hours wrestling with fear,

worry and hate. Win the war against these insidious scourges.

3. *Strengthen Your Self-Image.* See yourself as you've been in your best moments, and give yourself a little appreciation. Visualize your happy times and the pride you've felt in yourself. Imagine future experiences that will be joyful; give yourself credit for what you are. Stop beating your own brains in!

4. *Learn How to Laugh.* Adults sometimes grin or chuckle, but not many can really laugh. I mean a real belly laugh that gives one a sense of release and freedom. Laughing, when it's genuine, is purifying. It is part of your success mechanism, jet-propelling you to victories in life. If you haven't laughed since the age of 10 or 14, go back into the school of your mind and re-learn something you never should have forgotten.

5. *Dig Out Your Buried Treasures.* Don't let your talents and resources just die inside you; give them a chance to meet the test of life!

6. *Help Others.* Giving to your fellows can be the most rewarding experience of your life. Don't be cynical; understand that many people who seem unpleasant or hostile are wearing a facade that they think will protect them from others. If you give to others, you might be amazed at their grateful, appreciative response. Some people who seem the hardest are really soft and vulnerable. You'll feel great when you can give, without thought of profit.

7. *Seek Activities That Will Make You Happy.* Golf, tennis, water skiing? Painting, singing, sewing? I can't tell you—you'll have to tell yourself. But an active life is a happy life, if you're doing what's good for you and good for others.

How to Relax The Easy Way

If you're an office or desk worker or anyone who wants to relax but lack time, all you need is about 20 minutes for this easy Relax-Ercise. All you need is a chair *and concentration* to drain out of your body the stress and strain that makes you tense.

1. Sit on a chair, with both feet *squarely* on the floor. Rest lightly on the chair. Don't strain at it.

2. Imagine you weigh much more than you do. Where is all this heavy weight resting? Right on the chair. You are letting the chair hold it all up.

3. Take three deep breaths. Slowly fill and empty your lungs completely. If possible, do it before an open window where you can get bracing outdoor air.

4. Relieve the strain of your neck muscles by letting your head fall forward as if you have no stiffness in your neck at all. Imagine how your head would drop off your shoulders if it were not attached. *Then let it fall!*

5. Now relax your eyes by imagining that little weights have been attached to your eyelids. These weights close your eyelids. Try to lift them. Let them fall shut about three more times.

6. Relax your face muscles by letting them go limp. Relax further tension by raising your right arm very high above your head. Let it go completely limp, falling by its own weight onto your right knee. Repeat until you feel new strength coming into your arms. Do this 6-step exercise in just 20 minutes and relax your way to health.

Eat Relaxing Foods. Your foods should be mild and as natural as possible. Avoid sharp condiments and artificial flavors. Drink lots of mild raw vegetable juices. Much about how foods can help your nerves will be found in my book, *The Natural Way to Health Thru Controlled Fasting* which you can buy at the health food store.

Home Remedies For Relaxing

Comforting Heat is Soothing. Heat is soothing remedy for ironing out the kinks in your muscles. By dilating your blood vessels and increasing your circulation, it nourishes your body. Remember the old reliables: the hot water bottle, the tub bath, the electric pad, the infrared lamp.

How to Relax Your Eyes. To soothe the fatigue and strain in your eye muscles, to stimulate the circulation, try this easy remedy: apply a washcloth that has been soaked in lukewarm water to the closed eyes. Let the cloth remain for 5 minutes or until cool. Follow with an application of comfortably cool water to stimulate the eyes.

A Hot Foot Bath. Soak tired, aching feet in hot water for 15 or 20 minutes. Benefits include a stimulated circulation; the soak sends the blood tingling through the blood vessels and tension is relieved. A nervous person has cold feet or hands and the soak helps re-distribute the blood pressure.

Moist Heat Application. Soak a large bath towel in hot water, wring it out, place it on the tense, congested area (such as your neck and shoulders, small of your back, spine). To retain the heat longer, cover the towel with another dry towel, plus a small blanket over all this to keep the heat in. Just 15 minutes helps to relax the tight, tense muscles of your body.

Think Yourself To Relaxation. The noted clergyman, Dr. Joseph Murphy in *The Power Of Your Subconscious Mind,* tells us: "If you really want peace of mind and inner calm, you will get it. Regardless of how unjustly you have been treated, or how unfair the boss has been, or what a mean scoundrel someone has proved to be, all this makes no difference to you when you awaken to your mental and spiritual powers.

"You know what you want, and you will definitely refuse to let the thieves (thoughts) of hatred, anger, hostility and ill will rob you of peace, harmony, health and happiness. You cease to become upset by people, conditions, news and events by identifying your thoughts immediately with your aim in life."

What is that aim: RELAXATION! *Do it now!!*

EIGHT

BEAUTY TIPS

by

LINDA CLARK

—Light On Your Health Problems

HAIR

Q. Help! Help! I want to be beautiful, too, but between my office job and my home responsibilities, I don't have time. I can't even get to a hairdresser. Isn't there a simple routine I can follow?—A.T., New York City

A. The simplest natural beauty routine I have read for a long time was described in *Vogue,* in June, 1970. An actress told how she cares for her super-sheen, never-set, beautiful chestnut hair. She rubs in warmed olive oil and distributes it through her hair and on her scalp with a plastic scalp massager before shampooing twice weekly. She uses two soapings to remove the oil.

On her face she applies a formula from her grandmother: mix with a fork a raw egg, lemon juice and olive oil and spread on the face to remain for 10 minutes to help tighten pores.

She does her exercises in the bathtub where the warm water helps relax her muscles.

For her nutritional program she steams, not boils, her cooked vegetables, and juices her raw vegetables. For breakfast she puts in a blender orange juice, wheat germ, raw eggs and honey. This, she says, provides her energy.

When asked what makes a woman beautiful, she answered promptly, "Joy, feeling good, active and satisfied."

Such a program takes a minimum of time and should bring a maximum amount of beauty.

Q. My hair is so thin! How can I make it thicker, as it used to be?—B.P., Toledo, Ohio

A. I recently received a letter from a man who has done some further experimenting. He says: "My hair is growing back again. The male pattern baldness (shaped like a receding "M" above the forehead) is slowly going away. I have increased my protein intake, vitamin and mineral intake, use more carrot juice, etc. My supplements are mostly from natural sources. I work on my hair for one hour each day while watching TV—massaging not only the head, but the area from the neck up. My scalp is now loose, hair is growing fast, coming in on the sides and down the center. I have a long way to go but I see definite results. I brush and massage, brush and massage, to step up circulation to the scalp. I even discovered the rolling pin and use that for variety! I'm also using applications of vitamin E since a Japanese experiment states that it makes hair grow 2.4 times faster. This improvement of mine has taken 10 months but it is worth it, and still continuing."

Q. How much vitamin B-2 is safe to take? My 19-year-old granddaughter has unreasonably oily hair. One book says that 5 to 15 mg. will work for this problem, but it has not. She takes 20 mg. of B-2 daily, but has to wash her hair every day since she can almost squeeze the oil out of it. She eats a good diet.—J.C., Lamont, California

A. I cannot prescribe so I cannot say, nor do I know, how much vitamin B-2 your granddaughter needs, or if that is the entire problem. Each person differs. It is true that during the teens oil glands are overactive. Too frequent shampooing, and very hot water overstimulate these glands into secreting even more oil. If shampooing in medium warm water is extended to two days, then three days, and finally to a week apart, the oil glands usually slow down in their manufacture.

I called Jheri Redding on this question. His years in the natural beauty field are unsurpassed, and I (and thousands of beauty salons nationwide) have the greatest respect for his natural beauty knowledge. He advised, for this problem, using an acid-based shampoo (can be ordered by health stores) followed by an Ep-

som salt rinse. Dissolve 2 tablespoons of Epsom salts to
1 quart of warm water, he said. Towel dry the hair after shampoo and apply this rinse to the hair, but do not
wash it off. Set the hair; allow it to dry. Use the rinse
every third day, gradually extending it to once a week
until the condition improves.

*Q. Can dandruff or flaky scalp be caused by nervous-
ness? I take vitamin and mineral supplements daily, use
only organic shampoo and use little hair spray, but I do
tend to be a nervous person. Also, I would like to
know if a person can be allergic to the sun? Every time
I am exposed to the sun for even a short time, I break
out into itchy bumps. If this is an allergy, what can be
done to overcome it? I would like to be at least tanned
enough to look healthy.—S.L.S., Portland, Oregon.*

A. I checked with two physicians. Some people are definitely allergic to sun. Since you mention that you are a
nervous person, the physicians (they are both nutritional) wondered if you were getting enough foods and
natural supplements which provide B vitamins? I suggest you read and learn everything possible about the
entire B complex. The richest food sources are liver,
brewer's yeast and wheat germ. Supplements should
also include the *entire* B complex, and be derived from
nartual sources.

The skin and hair can certainly reflect a nervous
condition. If your skin responds, why not your scalp,
which is part of the skin system? Animals, as well as
people, are helped, also, with this dry, flaky condition
by taking more unsaturated oils in their diet. For good
balance in nutrition, be sure that you have ALL the
nutritional substances, not merely a few. Sometimes too
much of one B vitamin, for example, may cause a deficiency of another. You need the works!

Sun-worshipping, because it can cause an aging skin
as well as skin cancer in some individuals, is going out

of style. If you read up and take all the known nutrients, and eat nutritious foods, you should look healthy
without being tanned. You will also look younger longer.

*Q. Is there any danger in wearing a wig? My hair looks
so bad that it is the only solution I have found.*—T.O.,
Hollywood, California

A. One of the best answers to your questions I have
found comes from Lessie Caraway, who is the owner of
a beauty salon near Monterey, California. She says:

"A great danger signal is sweeping America today. I
feel we are standing unwisely by and watching the
women of this country lose all of their beauty by not
explaining to them what can happen to their hair when
they do not take proper care of it.

"I feel it will be a sad day when we see ⅔ of the
American women having to wear wigs the rest of their
lives. A woman should wear a wig, at the most, 3 days
a week, but I find women wearing wigs from 48 to 65
hours per week. This cannot go on for too long a time
without some permanent damage and that's when the
sad time will be. It makes no difference how strong
grass on a lawn might be. If you turn a pail down over
it and let it stay one month, it will kill the roots of the
grass.

"Well, the hair on the head is a little stronger than
that, but don't tell yourself you can wear a wig 10 and
12 hours a day. I feel it just won't work. I feel that if a
woman starts wearing a wig every day, 8 to 12 hours
per day, by the time she does this 8 to 10 years, the actual texture of her hair will change and diminish. I feel
if a woman begins wearing a wig steadily at the age of
23, by the time she is 35, her hair may have the appearance of an 80-year-old woman.

"One of the things to keep in mind is that people
who have studied and worked with wigs do not have a
collection of wigs themselves. As they learn about wigs,

they become acquainted with all the phases, good and bad, of wearing wigs too often."

Q. Is there any substitute for false eyelashes? They are so much trouble to apply.—G.C., Denver, Colorado

A. Yes. Emily Wilkins, in her book, *A New You* (a book for teen-agers, published by Putnam and Co.), suggests a method which can work for adults, too. She writes, "False eyelashes may cause your own eyelashes to fall out. Every time you glue them on and pull them off you are courting trouble. Instead, you can produce the look of false eyelashes with this method: Coat your lashes with mascara. Apply a little powder to the tips of the lashes with a cotton swab. Recoat with mascara. Repeat, if necessary. The result: fantastic, fluttery eyelashes."

FACE

Q. I am a dietitian. I would like to know what can be done for the prevention of whiteheads on the face. I have consulted specialists but none were able to answer. I am very anxious to know.—Mrs. F.U., Fort Lee, New Jersey

A. I went to my oracle of natural beauty, Jheri Redding, for help with this problem. This is what he said: A whitehead is sebaceous material which is caught by or in a membrane in the subcutaneous layer of the skin. Since it cannot come all the way through, it becomes a whitehead. To eliminate it, soften and deep cleanse the skin in order that this bit of sebaceous material can get all the way through—and off! To do this, Mr. Redding advises to keep the skin softened with any unsaturated vegetable oil, day and night for four or five days. This will soften the under cuticle and allow the whitehead to finally push through and be eliminated.

From then on, he added, keep your skin well cleansed to allow body oil and dirt to come through the pores easily. Taking vitamin C and E also has an effect on keeping the skin in a healthy condition in this problem.

Q. Is deep massage good for the face and neck?—B.L., Wichita, Kansas

A. A new book, *How to Use Your Hands to Help Your Face,* by Jessica Krane (Information Inc., New York, N.Y., 1969), states that heavy-handed massage can play havoc with your face. Miss Krane says rough or heavy massage will eventually break down the skin, tissues and musculature to the point that they can never be restored to normal. As a former concert pianist and a teacher of hundreds of classes of men and women in her method called "Face-o-Metrics," she advises a pianissimo (very soft) touch in smoothing cosmetics onto the skin. She feels that only gentle stroking relaxes the face so that lines seem to disappear of their own accord. She warns against touching the skin under your eyes with any pressure at all. "Leave it alone" she warns. Finger contact in cleansing or applying under eye make-up should be no heavier than a mere whisper, an art which must be learned.

Q. Is there a face exercise to plump out the cheeks and mouth of a person whose teeth have been pulled?—K.B., Granger, Washington

A. Any exercise which will bring fresh circulation to the face will help. Make a tight oval of the mouth and then try to stretch (while holding the oval) all the muscles of the face in a sunburst pattern outward and *away* from the oval. Several times night and morning will help the mouth and cheeks feel warm, showing that the circulation to those areas has been encouraged.

Nutrients help, too, as you will see in my book,

Secrets of Health and Beauty. Protein vegetable oils and lecithin added to the diet help to keep the tissues under the surface of the cheek and mouth area firm.

Q. I am going to be 69 soon. I have a pretty good skin for my age, but the thing that worries me most are the lines around my mouth. They make me very self-conscious. Is there anything I can do to make them disappear or appear less conspicuous? I do wear dentures, but so does my husband. Though he is older he doesn't have these wrinkles.—Mrs. O.C., Cleveland, Ohio

A. The lines around your mouth are no doubt due to poor muscle tone in that area, causing the tissues to shrink and wrinkle. This would indicate that these muscles need more protein. To plump them up from the inside, increase your protein intake via your diet, being sure that you have enough hydrochloric acid to help digest and utilize it. (This may well be the difference between you and your husband. Even though you eat the same diet, he may be assimilating his protein better than you).

Vitamin B-2 often helps this condition, too.

To plump up the tissues from the outside, apply the liquid collagenous protein for cosmetic purposes. To 3 oz. of any type of unsaturated vegetable oil, add 1 oz. of the protein. Stir before each use. Rub in and leave all night. Health stores can at last definitely get this collagenous protein.

Finally, use an exercise daily to help strengthen the muscles and tighten them so that the wrinkles will be helped to smooth out. Make an O with your mouth and tense *hard* several times until you feel all the area around your mouth tighten and fresh circulation warming it up.

HELP FOR SCOWL LINES

Q. Can you give me an exercise to reduce or eliminate a scowl line?—A.B., Columbus, Ohio

A. Marjorie Craig's book has an exercise for the scowl line. To lessen lines between the eyebrows, she says, "Start with eyes wide open, then pull brows down over the eyes in a real frown. Frown even harder; then lift the eyebrows as high as you can, at the same time opening your eyes as wide as you can. Frown-and-lift 5 times."

Another exercise is: Sit at a table or desk. Put your right elbow on the surface of the table or desk and then rest the frown area against the heel of your right hand. Now push the frown lines against the heel of your hand. Don't let the *hand* do the pushing; let the frown area push against your hand! This strengthens these face muscles themselves. After you have done this several times, then use compression. Here's how: Use the soft pads of your three middle finger tips. Press the frown area and let go. Press and let go. Do this several times. This compression method really brings the blood to the surface you wish to smooth and helps to plump up the skin at that point. Physiotherapists often use this method to bring fresh blood to a lazy or sluggish part of the body. But don't delude yourself that these exercises will cure unless you use prevention, too. Frowning is a habit and each time you frown it deepens the crease in your skin.

To help remember not to frown, as well as smooth away a frown line for a while, use Arlene Dahl's suggestion of putting Scotch magic tape on your frown area while you work or while you sleep. It's a real help.

Q. After an operation some years ago, my doctor prescribed some hormones which caused thick hair growth on my upper lip. This hair growth was removed

*by electrolysis, but probably weakened the muscles.
Consequently, deep vertical lines developed. Can anything be done to eliminate them?*—Miss A., New Or-
leans, Louisiana

A. There are two avenues to follow here: One, increase
the use of protein in your diet to help rebuild both skin
and muscles (skin is about 95 percent protein). The
other is to use a mouth exercise to strengthen the muscles in that area. Make an "O" with your lips. Holding
you cheeks and upper lip areas taut, make this "O" bigger and wider as if you were saying "Wow," against the
strong resistance of the entire lower part of your face.
You will feel the circulation increasing in these areas,
and thus the blood stream can help nourish and
strengthen the area you wish to improve.

*Q. I have been on a nutritional program for years. It
has included vitamins, minerals, fruits and raw vegetables. As I get older, my upper lip is getting wrinkles.
Why?*

Also, what is good exercise to reduce hips?—M.E.J.,
Atlanta, Georgia

A. You do not mention protein in your nutritional program. Not only is skin nearly 98% protein, but the muscles which support it are also made of protein. When
protein is undersupplied to the body, the results are not
noticeable at first, but flabbiness and wrinkles become
apparent as one ages and the deficiency increases. Adding protein to the diet to help regenerate the muscles
under your lip, and in other facial areas, and applying
protein in some form to the skin itself, will help. Collagenous protein liquid for skin and hair application is
becoming available in health stores. Read and follow
the directions.

One more thing: Place the fingertips of both hands
on your upper lip to hold it firm, then try to make a

wide "O," pulling inwards and outwards with your mouth against the resistance of your fingertips. Repeat several times to bring circulation to the lip area.

Debbie Drake suggests this exercise for hip reducing: Stand with your hands on your hips. Cross the right leg over the left knee and as you step forward, bend your knee as far as you can. Now cross the left leg over the right knee with another deep knee bend. Do this exercise as a walk, starting with a few steps and increasing the number each day. According to Debbie Drake, you will feel the pull as this firms, slims, shapes and trims the hips. She also suggests walking, stairclimbing, and bicycling for improving hips and thighs. Golf and tennis are means of having fun and improving your figure at the same time.

SKIN

Q. What causes large pores? What can I do to make them smaller?—Mrs. M.E.L., Cincinnati, Ohio

A. Large pores indicate a lack of tensile strength in the muscles around the pore itself. Two methods may be used to correct this condition: helping to rebuild the muscle by applying protein (of which muscle is made) and using a tightening substance as well. A liquid protein is available in some beauty salons and is also becoming available in health stores. This substance can be applied to the skin as a night treatment, according to the directions which accompany it. Witch hazel can be smoothed on during the daytime as a tightener. For faster results, rubbing your face with an ice cube or so, wrapped in a cloth, may help.

Above all, cleanse your face every eight hours! The debris that is constantly expelled through the skin (though invisible to you) should not be allowed to remain in the pores to stretch them.

Q. I have oily skin and tend to get enlarged pores, although I wash frequently and use an astringent. Is there anything else I can do to minimize this problem? Also, would you recommend the use of mayonnaise on the face (or hair) as described in your book, Secrets of Health and Beauty, *when the condition is so oily to begin with?*—W.H., Long Beach, California

A. I asked Jheri Redding, because of his many years of experience in the natural beauty field, for help with this question. Here is his answer: "Mix three parts of collagenous protein with one part of distilled water and apply as you would a cream. (This mixture should be refrigerated and will last for three weeks.)

"Research points to the fact that the addition of the B vitamins, particularly B-6, pantothenic acid as well as vitamin A taken daily, are extremely beneficial. It would be advisable to keep on using the mayonnaise as it is also beneficial for this condition."

Q. I am allergic to commercial deodorants and break out in a rash when I use them. Are there any available which do not contain the aluminum sulfate which I think is what causes my problem?—M.H., Kansas City, Missouri

A. You can find a deodorant at health stores which is free from this or other chemical additives, or watch the mail order ads for one which is so gentle that no one I know who has used it has had any unpleasant reaction. It contains no irritants at all. Chemically the active ingredients are from the borated soda family—making the deodorant cream effective and harmless. It can even be used on the hands to deodorize them after cutting onions!

Q. For a number of years I have been bothered with very dry skin on my lower lip only, with little flakes of the dry skin constantly forming, which makes the lip very rough. I have applied castor oil, wheat germ oil and many of the vegetable and seed oils from the health food stores with no results. Is there anything I can do to correct this condition?—J.K.R., Hollywood, California

A. I called on two experts in this field. One was Katie Pugh, author of *Hair Thru Diet,* as well as Jheri Redding, who knows so much about skin problems. I asked Katie because she mentions in her book that after using a photo-sensitive lipstick, her own lips peeled for two or three years. She said: "To heal the scalds and burns of the lipstick, I worked from the inside mostly. I took large amounts of B complex, plus extra B-2, plus other B complex any way I could get it, including liquid form. I also took natural oils. I used no lipstick for over three years. Just applying something on the lips never worked. I tried for months that way. It was only after the above routine that they healed. To keep the lips from cracking I used a natural lip pomade stick."

Jheri concurred with this approach. He also advocated vitamin B for the condition. And while I had him on the phone I asked what to do for hangnails. He advised vitamin E.

Q. I have ugly stretch marks on my breasts, hips and thighs as a result of an extensive weight loss. I acquired them three years ago. Is there anything I can take internally or apply externally to erase these marks?— L.S., Long Beach, California

A. Our grandmothers used cocoa butter (available in drug and some health stores). They rubbed it on their stretch marks which followed childbirth and the marks disappeared. Remember, too, that skin is about 97 per cent protein. If you are deficient in protein or in hydrochloric acid (which helps your body assimilate protein), adding both to your diet should help. Many people state that taking a heaping tablespoon of protein powder in juice once or twice daily, in addition to using protein at every meal, has helped them to become firm.

An anthropologist from the University of California, Dr. R. D. McCracken, recently told the American Anthropological Association that "man is basically a meat-and fruit-eating animal. The carbohydrate or starches are an unnatural diet for him. Carbohydrates make sugar more easily absorbed by the body and upset delicate body chemistries. Proteins are eventually converted to sugar but much more slowly and safely." Carbohydrates also tend to make one flabby, which can lead to loose skin.

Q. In the past five years many brown spots have appeared on the backs of my hands, and now are appearing on my face, high up on my cheeks. I have consulted several specialists but none have been able to give the cause or the remedy. I should appreciate any suggestions.—Mrs. J.N.M., Odessa, Texas

A. Quoting one expert, "You cannot have a clear skin if your intestines are clogged with poisons and toxins, which lead to a toxic liver. ... Brown spots on hands or face are merely a sign that poisons have piled up in the intestines and liver." The woman who made this statement has a beautiful, clear, pink-and-white skin.

Adelle Davis has said that taking vitamin E helps to fade spots in some (not all) people. Others advocate applying vitamin E or castor oil directly to the spots. I recently investigated an English product (not available yet in this country) which helped many people who rubbed it on the spots. The product contains sulfur.

EYES AND NAILS

Q. What can I do to lengthen and strengthen my fingernails?—V.W., Los Angeles, California

A. I have mentioned bone meal before. According to Alfred Aslander, Ph.D., of Sweden, this should be *true* bone meal, not bone ash, which he believes is not fit for human consumption. He says you can tell the difference easily: bone ash is chalk white, looks like chalk, but with no taste or odor. True bone meal, he says, is somewhat yellow in color and has a faint animal taste and odor. It contains more nutrients and minerals in addition to the calcium. People who take it regularly report stronger teeth, bones and fingernails.

Another help: a reader recently wrote me that she experienced the first real growth of fingernails in her lifetime as a result of eating a few fresh comfrey leaves daily. The leaves—if young—can be added to salads or if they are larger can be blended in a blender into a juice or health drink together with other ingredients of your choice.

Q. What causes fingernail ridges? I am 52 years old, teach school, and am under pressure and strain a lot. The ridges started several years ago.—O.G., Dallas, Texas

A. You did not say whether the ridges were horizontal or longitudinal. Horizontal ridges are formed during menstruation. Longitudinal ridges are a result of anemia. Be sure you include in your diet, liver (fresh or desiccated) and other natural sources of iron (ask your health store) as well as generous portions of protein, of which nails are largely made.

Q. I will soon be 50 and my eyelids are getting so baggy. What causes this? Can anything be done to keep them from getting worse? Do face exercises help?— Mrs. E., Miami, Florida

A. Marjorie Craig, in her book, *Miss Craig's Face Saving Exercises* (Random House, N.Y.C., November,

1970), gives a corrective exercise for this condition, which is no doubt due to weak muscles and perhaps too little protein. She advises: "Looking into a mirror, tightly place thumb and index finger on side corners of eyes. Close your eyes. Then squeeze the corners of your eyes in *toward your fingers* (first position). When you think you have squeezed as hard as you can, squeeze even harder (second position). S-l-o-w-l-y release the squeeze. Do the entire exercise three times.

Q. What causes dark circles under the eyes? How can I get rid of them?—E.H.J., Washington, D.C.

A. Dark circles can be caused by an allergy. This is often the case in people who are using a commercial hair dye or tint. Actually, since chemical in the hair dye (or even a cosmetic) may be the cause, the body, particularly the liver, needs help in detoxifying.

But there is another surprising cause of dark circles. I have never seen a person with a parasite (intestinal) infestation who did not have dark circles. In fact, in members of my own family who lived in India, where intestinal parasites are common, I have found a perfect correlation between dark circles and parasites. When the parasites were routed, the circles disappeared. Your doctor can make a test to see if you have them and give you the proper remedy.

Q. What can I do for very swollen, puffy eyelids on arising every morning? The swelling lasts for several hours, sometimes most of the day. I am in my late 40's and my doctor tells me I am in very good health.—Mrs. J.H., San Jose, California

A. Eye puffiness can come from excessive water retention, which, if your doctor has ruled out kidney disturbance, might yield to a natural diuretic, such as vitamin

B-6, vitamin C, or magnesium; or it can be caused by a deficiency of protein.

Most likely, though, you are suffering from an allergy. What do you put on your face the night before? Eliminate it and see if it does not disappear. It might even be an allergy to pillows, bedding or some environmental situation. Do a little detective work until you find, and eliminate, the culprit.

NINE

YOU AND
YOUR GLANDS

by

MELVIN E. PAGE, DDS & H. LEON ABRAMS

—Your Body Is Your Best Doctor

THE SECRETS to the inner workings of the body chemical laboratory are the glands. The body has numerous glands such as the sweat glands and salivary glands, but the master regulators of body metabolism are the endocrine glands. They are called endocrine glands because they empty their hormones directly into the blood stream. The blood stream then takes these hormones, which are chemical compounds manufactured in minute amounts, to the rest of the body and other glands. The glands work in harmony or unison. If one is malfunctioning, it will affect the others to a greater or lesser degree. Our endocrine glands not only take part in everything that we do, but actually make it possible for us to do what we do. They govern our temperament and, physiologically, our everyday activities. For example, lift your little toe or finger; it is vital hormones see to it that blood sugar is in the blood stream to feed the muscles so that muscle power is available. Cut your hand, or any part of your body, and hormones help to control inflammation and keep infection from setting in. These hormones may be described as tiny hydrogen bombs which are powerful almost beyond description. They circulate through the blood system, going to the right places and doing just the right things in a normally healthy body. But, when one group of hormones are in excess, deficient, or otherwise abnormal, they upset the entire glandular system with the result that the entire body mechanism and functions are out of order.

There are eight of the endocrine glands which taken all together weigh only approximately two ounces. Yet, this is probably the most important two ounces in the entire body. These glands function as a board of directors, council of ministers, and regulators of body chemistry. They work together, in a healthy situation, so harmoniously that if one is sluggish, another gives it a helping hand or can assume part of its function depending upon the circumstances. They are further subdivided into working groups. One of these functional

97

groups consists of the pineal-thymus sex glands. Similar functional group relations exist between the pituitary, thyroid and adrenal glands which are functionally connected with the sex glands. To understand these glands and their functions, it is necessary to take up each one separately.

The pituitary gland has been termed the most remarkable component of the human body because of its great influence on the other glands and may be said to be likened to the conductor of a symphony orchestra in reference to its relationship to the other glands. The pituitary is a double organ, the anterior pituitary and the posterior pituitary, which are separate glands. Together these two lobes are about the size of a large pea situated in the bony cavern on the underside of the brain at about the center of the head. The position of the pituitary gland, which gives it maximum protection, is indicative of its importance.

One of the most fascinating substances produced by the anterior pituitary gland is the growth hormone. It controls growth. An under-active anterior pituitary gland may not produce enough of this hormone for the individual to reach the maximum height to which he would ordinarily grow, and is responsible for dwarfism. Man has created some dwarfs purposely by inbreeding for very under-active anterior pituitary glands. An example of this is the dachshund dog which owes its dwarfed form to a considerable under-active pituitary gland.

Conversely, if the anterior pituitary gland is very much over-active in its production of the growth hormone, the result is a giant. Most circus giants are a result of a very abnormal over-activity. If the anterior pituitary gland grows larger in adult life, after one's skeleton has become set, parts of the skeleton may begin to grow again. Since the growth zones have become completely set, only the free ends of the bones of the chin, feet, nose, and hands can grow. This disease is known as acromegaly. It is the growth hormone from the anterior pituitary which prompts growth in a new born babe; it receives these human growth hormones from its mother's milk. Those who drink cow's milk get the cow growth hormone. That is why those who have an over-active anterior pituitary gland should not have milk after the weaning period. More will be said about this in the chapter on milk. An over-active anterior pituitary gland is often associated with cancer. It is easy to see this relationship when we realize that most of the types of cancer are really cells gone wild in their growth pattern. When the gland is over-active it is producing too much of the powerful growth hormone and it is bound to have its effect upon the other glands of the body and the cells. The importance of this gland can hardly be overly exaggerated when we realize that the anterior pituitary may be described as a kind of governor of all the other endocrine glands.

The pituitary gland plays a major part in the birth process. Following delivery of a baby it releases a very minute amount of a hormone which causes contraction of the mother's womb. This is one of nature's guards agaisnt excessive bleeding that can result in death. A few days following birth another hormone from the anterior pituitary, is released. It is one of the truly extraordinary chemicals ever discovered—prolactin—which stimulates the breast to produce milk and largely accounts for mother love. To judge from experimentation with animals, it seems most likely that individuals' ability to produce this hormone is responsible for their differing abilities to nurse babies and also in their attitude toward babies. All have observed that some women become natural mothers while others, if they perform their duties as good mothers, do it mainly because of social pressure.

The pituitary gland, along with the sex glands and the adrenal cortex, also plays quite an important part in sex. There certainly is no doubt that sex behavior is subject to all kinds of environmental influences, but to one who is familiar with endocrinology and biological variability, there is also no doubt that the glandular system, which is distinctive in each person, plays a major part in sex variability.

Another substance produced by the anterior pituitary is ACTH, the adrenocorticotropic hormone. It seems that this hormone has to do with disposition or general feeling of well-being. This indicates definitely that the hormonal differences of individuals may have a great deal to do with people's dispositions.

The posterior pituitary gland secretes hormones which help to control the salt and water balance of the body and control the gravity or density of the urine. If it were not for this control an individual would urinate as much as three gallons or more of urine a day.

When the posterior pituitary gland is not functioning properly one may be quite prone to diabetes insipidus, (excessive urination), arthritis, pyorrhea, high blood pressure, and other degenerative diseases depending upon how such a dysfunction affects the other glands and the body as a whole. An under-active posterior pituitary may be the reason for sterility in women.

From this little survey of the function of the pituitary gland it is easy to see that it is very complicated in both structure and function. The various parts manufacture many different hormones which themselves then interact with the other glands of the body in carrying out their special functions. As pointed out previously, these hormones are carried to all parts of the body through and by the blood stream. That is why the blood analysis is so important in any approach to body chemistry.

To a very considerable degree, our general well-being is dependent upon the speed at which our bodies live. The rate of speed of the basic cellular bodily processes is regulated by the thyroid gland. This gland is butterfly shaped and straddles the windpipe. It is approximately the size of a walnut. However, the size is dependent on many factors such as heredity, which determines whether or not it is normal or abnormal to begin with, and environment such as diet, which can greatly affect it. The thyroid gland has been likened to the accelerator of a car because it speeds up or slows down our body activities. The thyroid hormone determines whether the rate at which we live is in a slow, sluggish, sleepy, half-alive world or in an energy-charged, racing one. The hormonal production of a normal thyroid is only one twenty-eight-hundredths of an ounce per day (1/2800). When the gland produces too much hormone, that person is then said to have an over-active thyroid (hyperthyroidism) and when it produces too little, the individual has an under-active thyroid gland (hypothyroidism). When the gland is under-active it can cause the metabolism to slow down to such a subnormal level that the person may be said to be merely vegetating in his existence. When a person is suffering from an over-active thyroid gland, he is always in a rush and is the type that may be described as "burning the candle at both ends." Either one of these abnormal conditions, particularly when they become acute, can cause devastation to both body and mind. When one has an over-active thyroid, some of the symptoms which may be present are a ravenous appetite, pounding heart, and high blood pressure, and is likely to be very susceptible to ulcers and heart ailments associated with the nerves that control the heart.

With advancing age the thyroid often gradually tapers off its production of vital thyroid hormone. That is why many elderly people are said to have become cold natured in their advancing years. In these cases their bodies just are not producing enough heat. Sterility in some women is also due to an under-active thyroid which has slowed their bodily activities to such a degree that they are sterile.

The most commonly known disease of the thyroid

gland is goiter. This is just one of a number of degenerative diseases which may afflict it. Goiter may be associated with either an over-active thyroid or an underactive one. One of the major causes of goiter is due to a dietary deficiency of the mineral iodine. Iodine is extensively distributed in nature, but there are some parts of the world in which it is not present. People in these parts may suffer from an iodine deficiency. The natural way in which the body gets its iodine is from food, and sea foods.

An adult requires only 15 billionths of an ounce of iodine per day, but even that minute amount is not available in areas where iodine is deficient in the water, soil and plants, and therefore in the diet. An example of such areas are the Alps Mountain Regions of Europe and our own middle western states around the Great Lakes region. Today inorganic iodine is added to our table salt to guard against this deficiency. However, it is much healthier for the body to get its iodine in the natural form from foods. A healthy thyroid gland contains about four ten-thousandths 4/10,000) of an ounce of iodine. Other types of goiter are caused by other factors and have nothing to do with iodine.

Dr. Roger Williams, the outstanding biochemist of the University of Texas, who discovered one of the B vitamins, has stated that there are a great many people who are somewhat deficient in thyroid hormone and that they would be greatly benefited by taking a minute amount of it orally. However, these people do not usually feel sick enough to go to the doctor, so nothing is done about the situation. Still, it must be born in mind that the dosage must be minute and prescribed according to the individual patient's needs. Too much is just as harmful as too little.

The hormone manufactured by the thyroid gland is transported to the cells in a state of loose chemical combination with the globulin fraction of the proteins in the blood stream. In this condition the hormone can be taken from the blood for measurements of protein-bound iodine, which is generally referred to simply as a PBI blood test. This test is one of the most reliable for determining the amount of thyroid hormone circulating in the blood stream. In a normal person there should be a concentration of five to seven micrograms of protein-bound iodine per 100 cubic centimeters of blood, or five to seven parts per 100 million. When the thyroid is over-active the concentration often rises to 10 to 20 micrograms, whereas with an under-active thyroid it may go down to less than one microgram. The PBI test is one of the many tests used in our thorough and extensive blood analyses in determining the condition of one's body chemistry.

The parathyroids, four little glands about the size of little wheat grains, are situated alongside the thyroid. The main function of the hormone produced by the parathyroids is that of regulating the blood calcium level. They determine the transport of calcium from the bones into the bloodstream, body tissues, and see that excess calcium is thrown out in the urine. The calcium we get through our food, is first deposited in the bones (this is also controlled by other hormones) and later taken to the blood as the body requires. Of course, the parathyroids are in turn largely regulated by the other glands, but when the parathyroid hormone is deficient or lacking the body does not have enough calcium. One disease associated with calcium deficiency is pyorrhea; another is tetany, a condition in which the muscles twitch and spasms often appear. Calcium also inhibits the neuromuscular irritability of the body tissues. When there is too much calcium in the body it may result in arthritic deposits, kidney stones, and cataracts. How the calcium is utilized depends upon one's body chemistry.

The adrenals are little yellowish-brown glands which sit atop the kidney. We can get something of their importance when it is realized that each minute they receive six times their own weight in blood. The adrenals consist of two major parts and may be likened to a walnut. The kernel, which consists of nerve cells, is called the medulla, and the shell is called the cortex. These two parts of the adrenal glands produce remarkable and very powerful hormones.

Adrenalin is secreted by the kernel of the adrenals. Due to its part in preparing us for emergencies, adrenalin may be termed the "fight or flee" hormone. For example, a man who himself has been injured, rushes into a burning house and rushes out carrying the refrigerator, and then collapses. It was adrenalin that provided such a great spurt of power and strength. In times of great stress or danger, the hormonal production of adrenalin may suddenly shoot up to ten times the normal level, with the result that the heart and breathing rates increase while the level of energizing blood sugar shoots up. The normal level of adrenalin in the blood stream ranges from one two-billionth to two one-billionths, so you can see that it takes only the tiniest amount, even for the greatest emergencies. In that the adrenals cannot be sure how a conflict will come out, they also greatly quicken the clotting time of blood so as to reduce the loss of blood if one is cut. It is also adrenalin that acts as an oxidative ferment during nerve-cell activity, dilates the pupils of the eyes, contracts the capillaries, raises blood pressure, mobilizes sugar from the liver, increases the tonus of the heart muscles, and seems to play some part in the formation of skin pigmentation.

The adrenal cortex, the shell of the adrenals, manufactures a large number of different hormones or hormone-like chemicals; at present some 28 have been identified of which one is a sex hormone. Some of the body functions influenced by the adrenal cortex are mineral levels in the blood stream, carbohydrate metabolism, kidney function, the ability of muscles to respond to stimulation, stimulation of the sex glands, and resistance to stress caused by such things as bacterial poisons, too much insulin and thyroid hormone. Now substances similar to the adrenal cortex hormone are produced synthetically, such as cortisone. These were at first hailed as wonder cures for arthritis and many other diseases, but their use in very large doses has also proven to be something of a curse. Once again it is re-iterated that too much of the endocrine hormones are just as bad as too little. In most all of the cases that I have seen, the patient would have been much better off to have never taken cortisone.

Little is known about the pineal and thymus glands. The pineal gland may restrain the action of the sex glands while the thymus seems to play a part in the maturing process from childhood to adulthood. When adulthood has been reached, the thymus dries up and shrinks to only a small part of its former size.

The isles of Langerhans of the pancreas produce insulin. When insulin is not produced, the disease of diabetes is present. This is known as hypoinsulinism. People can be born with this condition or a tendency for it or it may develop due to the use of too much sugar. Insulin is carried by the blood stream to the muscles and the liver, whereby these organs are then able to utilize the sugar in the blood and to store it in the form of glycogen. Many people suffer from an under-active production of insulin, but unfortunately they do not recognize such until the situation has manifested itself seriously.

However, too much insulin is also very harmful. When the pancreas produces too much insulin, the condition is referred to as hyperinsulinism. Too much insulin in the system produces a low blood sugar. This is shown in the following symptoms: fainting or dizzy spells, ravenous appetite and general weakness. Whenever there is over-production of insulin it may be accompanied by an under-production of the anterior pituitary gland, the opponent of the isles of Langerhans. The anterior pituitary produces hormones which convert glycogen (stored body sugar) to usable sugar and puts it into the blood stream. One of the most important functions of insulin is that of fighting infection. Quite often people who constantly suffer from one type of infection or another suffer from having too little insulin. Insulin plays many parts other than in just preventing diabetes, but most people only associate its use with diabetes. A minute dosage of insulin is often all that many patients need to get their body chemistry functioning to its normal healthy level. It should be added also that a faulty diet, particularly sugar, is one of the foods which is definitely injurious to the insulin producing pancreas.

The sex glands are exceptionally important because they produce vital hormones which are necessary for a balanced body chemistry. The male sex glands, known as testes, produce the male hormone testosterone. This is an androgen. Both males and females need this hormone, but naturally men produce more than the female—it is the so-called masculine hormone. When a person produces too much androgen, that individual is characterized as being andric—in other words too male from the hormonal or glandular viewpoint. This is manifest in personality also; andrics are go-getters, they drive themselves too much, just as do those with an over-active thyroid. One sign of andricity is baldness, and andrics are likely to be much more subject to ulcers, cancer, heart or circulatory diseases. Andric men are especially prone to have prostate gland trouble.

The female sex glands, termed ovaries, produce the hormone estrogen in extremely minute quantities. During a woman's 30 childbearing years, she produces an amount of estrogen hormones approximately the weight of a postage stamp. At the time of puberty it takes only a very minute amount of estrogen to bring about such a change, the amount being approximately equal to only one little corner of a postage stamp. Individuals producing too much estrogen are termed gynics. Gynics are usually more of a submissive type of person. In order to be normal and healthy, men also must have a very minute amount of estrogen. Not enough estrogen may result in rendering one more susceptible to heart and circulatory diseases, nervous disorders, and mental disturbances. However, too much is also very harmful.

The term gynic is used to designate the condition of over-production of estrogen while the term andric is employed for the condition of over-production of testosterone or progesterone. In using the terms andricity and gynicity, it should be pointed out that this in no way has to do with sexual perversion or homosexuality. It refers to the production and function of the sex hormones in the human body. Each individual must have the proper balance of them to have good body chemistry and good health. Men and women must have a certain amount of both male and female hormones; naturally each sex requires more of its own sex hormone than that of the opposite sex, but both must be present in the proper amount to insure that the glands function properly. So, when it is said that a woman is andric, it does not mean that she is masculine. It merely means that she has an over-producing of androgens and is thus in an unhealthy situation, manifesting personality traits, which may make it very difficult for her to get along with her husband, if he is also andric. Likewise, when a man is gynic it does not mean that he is feminine, but that he has too high a production of estrogen and is thus likely to have a slower metabolism than normal, which also presents itself in personality or disposition. Two gynics of opposite sex are not apt to get along together very well either. However, when an andric and gynic marry they usually get along very well, particularly during the childbearing period. Nature has that way of taking care of future generations. In this case with an andric and gynic marrying, both of whom are abnormal in their andric-gynic balance, nature plays its part by seeing that at least a certain percentage of the children from this marriage will have a chance of being born with normal glandular patterns. You often hear it said that opposites attract, and this is one of the explanations for that. Of course, the ideal is for two people to both have perfect glandular balance. This is where your blueprint of construction comes in; it tells the story. Now, it does not mean that the situation is hopeless. By taking glandular supplement and following the diet along with understanding of the problem, the parties concerned can be made compatible.

In this approach to good health, it is easy to see what is done when a gland is under-active. You merely give the proper amount of that gland's hormone to the patient. But, what about the gland that is over-active. We have two divisions of the glandular system, the build-up glands, which are isles of Langerhans of the pancreas, posterior pituitary, parathyroid and adrenal cortex and female hormone, and the breakdown glands, which are made up of the thyroid, anterior pituitary, adrenal medulla and andric hormones. These two sets of glands are opposed to each other. For example, when the thyroid is over-active, the secretion from the pancreas may lower it. In other words each gland has its opposite or opposites which will inhibit its action. When the glands are functioning normally, glandular balance has been established. Glandular imbalance lies at the root of most, if not all, degenerative diseases.

Your blueprint of construction tells the glandular pattern with which you were born, but it does not tell what has happened to your glands since you were born. Thus further diagnosis becomes necessary and the tools here are extensive blood analysis, urine analysis, and blood pressure readings. As you have seen above, it is the blood that carries the glandular hormones to the various parts of the body and it is hormones themselves which determine the constituency of the blood.

All the tests are exceptionally important, but the major ones for a general index to efficiency of body chemistry are the calcium-phosphorus and blood sugar levels. During my 40 years of practice and research with many thousands of cases, it has been determined that the proper level of calcium-phosphorus is two and one-half parts calcium to one part phosphorus. The blood sugar level should be exactly 100 milligrams of blood sugar per 100 cubic centimeters of blood. The endocrine glands which participate in one way or another upon blood sugar levels are the isles of Langerhans of the pancreas, anterior pituitary, adrenals, the thyroid and the sex glands. From all this you can see that there is a complicated process of inter-action of these glands. For example, over-activity of the anterior pituitary may lead to a high blood sugar level, whereas under-activity of the isles of Langerhans can produce the same effect. Low or high blood sugar levels in turn affect the calcium-phosphorus level of the blood. We have already seen what the effects of too much or too little calcium may be. Excessive phosphorus is also dangerous, it may cause headaches, nausea, yellow skin, weariness, and inflammatory conditions which may show up anywhere in the body. Certainly when the cholesterol level is too high the glands are not working properly. The cholesterol level actually has little to do with diet but is dependent upon proper glandular functions and is only indirectly influenced by diet as such influences the glands. Too high or too low a cell volume informs the doctor that something is wrong, and so it goes with each one of the analyses made.

It cannot be emphasized too much that the use of endocrine hormones in treatment to bring about good body chemistry must be used in very minute amounts which vary with each patient.

In dealing with people, no two of whom are indentical, each person must be dealt with as an individual. One cannot prescribe that everyone suffering from a specific degenerative disease, such as heart attacks, should receive the same amount of the same hormone or even the same treatment. The dosage that is just right for one person may be undesirable for another, but when used in the proper amount the results are as desired. Hormones keep our bodies functioning properly, or improperly, depending upon whether or not glandular balance is present. The body chemistry approach is to establish what is needed for each individual for his specific needs. In other words, the body chemistry approach to good health treats the whole person as an individual, not just the disease. When good body chemistry has been established, and is maintained, there should be no premature degeneration. With maximum chemical efficiency each individual should then be expected to live the whole life span with which he was endowed by God and nature in a normal healthy state of well-being.

FEEDING
THE PRE—SCHOOLER

by

GENA LARSON

—Better Foods For Better Babies

IN FEEDING the pre-schooler we want to remember that food has more meaning in child growth and development than simply as a nutrient to permit growth and maintenance. Food serves an equally significant role in at least three areas of development.

> *Physically*—In motor mastery of the body, eye, hand and mouth coordination, the complexities of swallowing and safe use of the mouth and throat muscles; in practice for future feeding and speech.
> *Mentally*—Feeding is a potent learning process. The child puts everything in his mouth, not with the intention of eating everything he finds, but of learning about everything within mouth reach through the sound, taste, and feel perceived through the mouth.
> *Emotionally*—Feeding is the primary interpersonal relationship with other people all through life. The infant learns about loving and being loved as he is nursed or held in his mother's arms to be fed.

Meal time for the pre-schooler should continue to be a pleasant time. Keep the servings small and, at least in the early months, offer just one food at a time in an unbreakable dish. Give him more of any food he enjoys and asks for, but don't coax or try to get him to eat more than he wants. No child ever starved himself to death!

Infant growth is so rapid and spectacular that many times we are ill-prepared for the slower changes of the second and third year, and many times we try to press food on the child in an attempt to continue the large appetite and rapid rate of growth of the first year.

We need to understand the difference between "poor" and "small" appetite. Do not be so dismayed by the small quantity of food eaten that you offer all manner of nutritionally poor or even "junk" foods, just to

113

get the child to eat something. Special care in the offering of high quality foods should be the rule.

Never allow your little ones to have carbonated drinks, candy or other harmful foods. What these "junk" foods do to the teeth is bad enough but what they do to the body and its vital functions is worse!

Be stern and firm with fond relatives or friends who come bearing gifts of candy, cookies or other "non" foods. Tell them your child's "tummy" is just barely big enough to hold all the *good* foods you want him to have.

A word here about illness. The pre-schooler often has many illnesses which are not a reflection on his care, but are due to his first encounters with communicable diseases.

Many times, the best food for a child is none at all. At the first sign of any illness, fever, sore throat, etc., *all* food should be withheld and only pure water should be given for a day or two. Fasting allows the body resources to work on the healing processes; energy used to digest and assimilate food hampers recovery. The child will have no appetite anyway but will require, instead of food: rest, sleep, peace and quiet, fresh air, and if the weather is nice, sunshine. These are nature's greatest healers, and they will often take care of simple illnesses without recourse to health-depleting shots and antibiotics.

Another thing we should remember is that some of the best childhood nutrition has probably been given in the form of small, frequent and wholesome feeding, while mother is preparing the family meals. Peas fresh from the pod, raw potatoes or carrots, bites of apples, raisins, or other raw fruits or vegetables will provide better quality nutrition than the finished cooked product at the dinner table. Food eaten with the fingers in happy companionship at mother's knee is good food.

Many pre-schoolers do well with a small, planned fourth meal at bedtime.

Do not be discouraged if your child does not learn at once to eat the good foods you would like him to eat. You came into the world with no food tastes developed. Remember you *learned* to like everything you enjoy now. Many mothers have a sad time trying to teach their youngsters to eat very bad foods.

Continue the codliver oil every day. The vegetables and fruits you prepare need not be grated or chopped as finely as for the younger child. You can now offer two kinds of food at once most of the time.

For a special breakfast treat, try a whole-grain or buckwheat yeast-raised pancake. It can be topped with butter and raw applesauce or a small amount of honey. Serve a small cup of milk or nut-milk if desired.

Lunch might include a green "finger" salad, homemade vegetable soup, a small serving of cottage cheese and milk. Other times serve banana pudding and yogurt or fresh fruit diced and a cube of natural raw cheese.

Dinner is much the same as lunch. Carrot-pineapple (or other) grated salad, a lightly cooked or raw green leafy vegetable or a yellow vegetable, or a baked potato with yogurt. Fish, meat or cottage cheese—a small serving.

Desserts should be fruit most of the time with an occasional "jellied custard" or a brown rice or millet pudding. Homemade ice cream is a special treat. Yogurt topped with fresh fruit is a festive dessert too and most youngsters enjoy a carob pudding once in a while.

Milk or yogurt may serve as a little bedtime snack, if one is desired.

Always use 100% whole grain in bread, cookies, pie crust, hot or cold cereal and add extra wheat germ or soy flour.

Use only natural sweeteners such as raw honey, honey comb, molasses, sorghum, date sugar, real maple syrup, dried fruits and carob powder.

For the child four years and older, raw nuts may be soaked overnight in milk or pineapple juice and served with fruit or green salads.

Sunflower seeds and pumpkin seeds are just the right size for tiny fingers. My grandchildren like to mix raisins with them or cut up date-bits and raw sesame seeds. These are great to take along in individual waxed bags on hikes or on camping trips. Celery may be stuffed with peanut or other nut butters or sesame cheese spread.

SUPER-SNACKS OR MEALTIME TREATS

Food offered as between-meal snacks should be high in quality and considered part of the daily nutrition. Most children will enjoy the following:

Honeycomb: instead of chewing gum. This is one of the richest known sources of the unsaturated fatty acids. It is to be chewed and enjoyed, then *swallowed;* the comb is perfectly digestible.

Popcorn: with raw butter or butter oil spread and sea salt.

Homemade ice cream or *fruit sherbets:* fruit and yogurt popsicles are delicious.

Celery: stuff with sesame cheese spread or any nut butter.

Partly toasted nuts or seeds: Place ⅓ cup seeds or nuts on a cookie sheet and toast in a 250° oven until golden brown. Place at once in a jar with a tight lid. Add ⅔ cup raw seeds or nuts. Cover and shake a bit to mix well. Let stand for a few hours at room temperature and all the nuts or seeds will taste toasted.

Gelatin desserts: Fruit juices made into gelatin desserts, and molded in a tube cake pan, make a pretty birthday cake for the little one. Top with honey sweetened whipped cream and candles.

Birthday watermelon: Cut the melon in half lengthwise. Trim a thin slice from the rounded side, so the melon will sit on a platter or tray. Press the candles into the fruit in any pattern. Good for older children too; just get a bigger melon.

Sardines: Many dentists recommend the regular use of canned sardines in the child's diet. The small edible bones seem to provide calcium and other minerals to help developing teeth. A small mound of freshly prepared sweet potato or white potato topped with sweet butter, and two or three tiny sardines, make a fine lunch. Most children consider sardines finger foods. Most mothers do not.

Beverages: The best beverages for the growing child are the ones already part of his mealtimes. Milk—plain or with a teaspoon of molasses and a half teaspoon of brewer's yeast for a special treat. Raw fruit or vegetable juices, or juices canned without added sugar. Read the label carefully. Frozen juices are usually better suited to the child's needs. Here again, purchase pure fruit juices, not the ones labeled "juice drinks." Home-canned fruit and vegetable juices are fine for baby too, especially if you grow your own poison-free foods or can purchase them in your area.

Salad sandwiches: Place a slice of raw cheddar or jack cheese between slices of zucchini or turnip. Spread apple or pear wedges with peanut butter or sesame cheese spread. Roll lettuce leaf up with cottage cheese filling. Finger lengths of celery may be stuffed with mixed peanut butter and cottage cheese. Slices of raw vegetables such as cucumber, turnip or zucchini may be cut in special shapes—stars, bells or Christmas trees, numbers, or letters (of the child's name etc.). Top with a dab of mashed avocado or nut butter.

Calf's heart: Buy calf's heart; wash, slice crosswise into rounds. Broil lightly on each side, or have your butcher grind beef heart into hamburger meat (⅓ heart, ⅔ beef): add egg and seasoning and shape into patties for broiling.

Frozen bananas: Bananas, cut in half crosswise and

frozen on a stick, are very good. Place on a cookie sheet lined with waxed paper to freeze. Dip in melted carob bar for an extra special treat. You can buy the wooden sticks in the paper goods section of your department store.

Avocados: Although classed as a fruit, the avocado provides more energy and nutrients, pound for pound, than almost any other food. Its digestibility approaches that of whole raw milk. Many minerals and the vitamins A, B, C, D, E and K are all contained in this blessed fruit. A good quantity of a high quality protein and a naturally unsaturated fat lie safe and protected within its unsprayed green covering. They are bland enough to blend with other flavors but have a delightful flavor of their own.

Mash and pile on a baked potato or use as a dip with carrot and celery sticks. Spread on small fingers of whole grain bread or toast. Dice and serve with a toothpick for a handy "spear," or dilute with milk for an instant avocado cream soup. Add a drizzle of honey and a bit of fruit juice or purée to the mashed avocado and there is dessert! Surely this fine natural food should be served often in the menu of both the child and adult.

> NOTE: Purchase the fruit hard and green at your market and place in a dark, warm place to ripen. It is spoon-ready when the fruit yields to gentle pressure between the palms of the hands.

Beets: Baby beets lightly steamed and served on a toothpick are easy to eat. Raw baby beets can be served as finger foods. Just don't watch!

Pushers: Tiny raw asparagus spears, or sturdy stalks of chard or kale, make fine edible "pushers" to help get other food onto the fork or spoon.

Pineapple tidbits: Cut fresh pineapple into one-inch squares. Dip in honey, then in crushed nuts or shredded coconut. Freeze until ready to serve. Bananas may be sliced in one-inch sections and served as above.

HELPFUL SUGGESTIONS

Fruits—Vegetables: Obtain organically grown fruits and vegetables as often as possible, or grow your own. When necessary to use commercially grown varieties, add a good vitamin-mineral supplement to the child's diet.

Supplementary amounts of vitamins E or A: To help a child take supplementary amounts of vitamins A or E, open a capsule with a needle, pour into a spoon of honeycomb or honey; mix well and serve. You may use this method for wheat germ oil also.

Cod liver oil: Cod liver oil is easy to take from a spoon. Have oil and spoon ice cold, in refrigerator. Follow with a swallow of milk or juice.

Pure water: Be sure your supply of water is safe and free of nitrates. Baby's tiny liver cannot detoxify chemicals or poisons as well as a grown-up liver can. If in doubt, have water tested by the Health Department.

Between-meal snacking: No eating between meals, except for small meals planned as part of the daily nutrition, or on Super-Special occasions. The mouth needs to remain empty for periods of three to four hours at a time, so the natural acids in the saliva can cleanse and protect the teeth.

How much is enough? Give your little chow hound as much or as little whole grain cereal, as much or as little fruit or vegetable or as much or as little yogurt, cottage cheese, egg or meat as he enjoys eating. Some days he will eat anything and everything; then there will be meals—even whole days—when he will mysteriously refuse to eat any or all of his foods. He may say to you, as my youngest granddaughter said to me recently, "I *can't* like applesauce this morning, Nana." Learn to respect his judgment and to remove the food promptly. Sometimes he may be cutting teeth or just not feeling up to par. When he has finished what he will eat willingly, take him out of the high-chair, without comment, not to *see* food again until the next mealtime.

WARNING: Keep all detergents, bleach, paints, poison sprays, cleaners, turpentine, aspirin and other medicines safely out of reach of your toddler. To a baby, *everything* that can be opened is to *eat* or *drink* and enough of a harmful substance can go down that tender gullet in one exploratory gulp to do drastic harm. Each year hundreds of children die from drinking or eating such substances. Do *not* leave your baby near such items even for a moment while you answer the telephone, go to the door, or turn the fire out under a kettle on the stove. Take the baby with you or place the object well out of reach. Do not give your baby aspirin or "baby aspirin," except under the supervision of your doctor. Many young children and babies die each year from an accidental overdose of this drug.

Car, air or sea sickness: If your child is troubled with "car sickness" or "air sickness," many mothers have found that this can be prevented if the child's diet is adequately supplied with vitamin B^6. To use, crush and dissolve a 25 milligram tablet of B^6 in water. Add to juice or other beverage before starting to travel. Foods containing B^6 are: heart, kidney, brewer's yeast, honey, egg yolk, cabbage and pecans. If more of these foods are included in your child's diet daily, this troublesome illness may never occur. Of course if *extra* B^6 is given, you must make doubly sure that all the other parts of the B complex are well supplied, otherwise a deficiency may be created. A little brewer's yeast may be stirred into the juice *with* the extra B^6, then all the other parts of the B vitamin "family" will be taken at the same time.

The mind needs feeding too! Everything said to a child, from the moment of birth, is registered in the little one's brain. Words of love, encouragement, praise and appreciation bring delight and joy to your child, long before he actually *knows* the meaning of such words. So let your praise be lavish, your words of love unlimited. Appreciate, out loud, each new accomplishment, each lesson learned. If your baby *knows* that you think he is a pretty fine fellow, he will quite likely grow up thinking you are right.

IN CONCLUSION

The most important part of eating to a child is the warm social interchange. To him the nutritional aspect of food is secondary. With a cheerful, unhurried mother and a contented child, mealtime can be what it should be—the happiest time of the day. Relax and enjoy your precious child. Love him a lot and do the best you can, knowing that food served with affection and care will do wonders while you are learning to do better.

ELEVEN

SOME BLENDER-MADE DISHES . . . MADE THE NATURAL WAY

by

FRIEDA NUSZ

—The Natural Foods Cookbook

MAGIC MILKS

I want to introduce you to magic-mix milks. These substitutes can be used in any recipe asking for milk. They are white as are other milks.

No. 1

3 eggs, raw or cooked
½ cup oil

Turn blender on and keep adding water gradually. When blender is full, pour into a jar and add water to make about 4½ to 5 cups of milk.

No. 2

½ cup sunflower seeds
½ cup sesame seeds
3 cooked eggs

Add hot water gradually until thick and smooth. Keep adding water to thin and when blender is full, pour into jar and add enough water to make 4 or 5 cups of milk. Sunflower alone is the mildest tasting. Use all sunflower seeds for sunflower-seed milk.

No. 3

1 cooked egg
¼ cup oil
⅓ cup water
⅓ cup brown rice, cooked

Blend until smooth. Add water to make 2 cups of milk. This is the closest to cow's milk that I think it's possible to come. This one is given in a smaller quantity to get the rice blended well. It can be strained through a small fine strainer to get it perfectly smooth. This one won't separate as fast as the other two. They all can be used in coffee to get the same taste as cream but will not look the same.

The eggs can be cooked in part of the water and added to the blender if you don't want to bother with cooking them in the shell.

These milks will sour at about the same rate as cow's milk.

DAIRYLESS MILK SHAKES USING FROZEN SWEETENED FRUIT
(thawed only enough to get it out of the package and broken up)

In blender:

    1 whole egg or two egg yolks
    ½ cup honey
    ½ cup oil
    1 teaspoon vanilla

Blend well and add approximately 1 cup of frozen presweetened fruit and approximately 1 tray of ice cubes. By using frozen fruit it will get very thick, almost like ice cream, so help turn on the top to make it easier for the blender and to help all the ice and frozen fruit to blend well. Can be gotten thick enough to eat with the spoon like ice cream.

Strawberry is the smoothest and tastiest. Raspberry has the fine seeds in it, but is also very good.

POTATO SOUP

Blend the potatoes until smooth in the blender with some of the cooking water. Blend the amount you want. For a smoother blend do not overload the blender; use about a cupful at a time. Pour into a saucepan. Now put in the blender any vegetables you have on hand—celery, parsley, carrots, green pepper and so on. Add enough water to blend these smooth and very fine.

Mix into the hot potato mixture. Add some browned hamburger, seasoning, and you have a delicious soup with the vegetables still raw. But cooked vegetables can be used too and blended in, or they can be cooked right with the potatoes and blended all at once. Add your favorite spices or onions. Onions are very good with potato soup. The onions can be browned in with the hamburger.

INSTANT SOUPS

Use any hot broth and add your raw vegetables. Chop or blend as fine as you like, and thin with more hot broth to taste, also season to taste with your favorite vegetable seasoning. This keeps your vegetables raw, but has a cooked taste and consistency. (Parsley is almost a must for good flavor in this kind of soup.)

CRANBERRY RELISH OR JAM

This cranberry relish or jell is different. Boil slowly 1 cup honey with one box of pectin powder. Add ½ cup of whole cranberries and boil slowly for about 10 minutes. Chop up 1½ cups raw cranberries in the blender and add to the surejell after it has boiled. Chill.

This makes a good jelly for using up any chopped fruit. Good with sour cherries too. Good with meat.

BLENDER CATSUP

1 quart drained tomatoes
¾ cup each Spice Vinegar and honey
1 teaspoon seasoning salt
¾ teaspoon celery seed

Onion salt to taste or a little raw onion blended in. Have blender running and drop in tasting, a little at a time, until it's the way you want it. Onion can be omitted. Refrigerate.

COLD GELATIN CHICKEN LOAF

You probably have bought a cold meat in the meat department of your market called turkey loaf? Well make an even better one with a stewing hen. Sliced thin, it's got a clear gel with white and dark pieces of meat throughout it. Cook one chicken with giblets in 1 quart of water until soft and easily removed from the bones. When cool, remove from the bones, and discard the ribs, neck, etc., to avoid getting a fine bone in the loaf. Add 5 or 6 tablespoons plain gelatin to the cool broth and allow to soften. Heat only long enough to melt the gelatin. Lay the chicken meat and giblet pieces in strips the long way in a loaf pan or square freezer container. When you slice it, the pieces will cut crossways and form little cubes in the slice. Refrigerate until set hard. Don't bother to skim any fat off before it is set, as it all rises to the top and can be washed off the stiff loaf under the hot water faucet. Unmold the loaf and it is ready for slicing. Season to taste with vegetable seasoning.

PANCAKES

(using whole grain)

Blend:
      1 cup whole kernels, with
      1 cup of milk or water,

Then add:
      ½ cup oil
      3 eggs
      1 tablespoon baking powder

Bake on hot griddle or pan, using butter with the first one to prevent sticking.

For waffles: Separate the eggs, using the yolks in the blender and beating the whites very stiff. Add the baking powder to the egg whites and pour the blender mixture over, folding it in.

If you don't want to use baking powder, they get good without it by beating the egg whites stiff separately. This goes for breads and muffins too. Either one of these two recipes can be used for muffins. Using baking powder will make a lighter, higher product.

When baking pancakes, where you beat the egg whites separately, give the center plenty of time to bake through before turning them over. They need a longer baking time to set the center. Don't have the heat too high, because they will brown too fast and be raw on the inside.

Milk makes a better bodied product than water; but to convert recipes using milk to dairyless, use ¾ cup water and another egg in place of 1 cup milk.

MIX-ME-QUICK CAKE

In blender:
    3 eggs
    ¾ cup honey
    1 teaspoon pure vanilla
    ¼ teaspoon pure almond
In bowl:
    1 cup of any flour (unsifted)
    ¾ cup oil
    1 tablespoon baking powder
Add in the order given. Pour blended mixture over dry ingredients in bowl; stir well. Bake all cakes at 325° to 350° till done. It's better to bake them slower and longer than at a high heat. If the bottom gets too dark, it spoils the flavor and they loose their moistness.

When using carob, use only vanilla flavoring.

When adding fruit, such as raisins, to the blender, you might not want to add flavorings to bring out the flavor of the fruit.

BONE MEAL COOKIES FOR BABIES
(Soft)

2 eggs
1 cup pitted dates, blend smooth
½ cup oil
Pour in bowl; add:
3 tablespoons carob
1 cup bone meal powder
Bake at 325° until done or set. Eating one per day is enough.

CHEESE CAKE

Since home-made cottage cheese varies in dryness, I'll give you the method instead of precise recipes.

Fill blender about half full with cottage cheese and turn on. Add milk until it's nice and smooth. Now to make it stiff when it's cold, add either one-half cup of melted butter to the running blender or a teaspoon of gelatin melted in a little hot milk. Add honey and vanilla and almond flavorings to taste. It doesn't take much honey because milk has a natural sweetness.

Variations for above

Drain a can of crushed pineapple or your own canned pineapple. Use the juice for blending the cheese and stir the pineapple into the batter. Pour into pyrex pan and chill. Or stiffen a can of crushed pineapple with a teaspoon of gelatin. Set a layer of this on the bottom or top of the cheesecake.

Pour on a crumb crust. Top with cinnamon.

BANANA PUDDING
(A Sweet No Sweets)

Blend:

> 3 cooked eggs
> 1 cup water
> ½ cup oil
> 3 bananas

Stir in 1 cut up banana in bowl or on top of pie. This is thick enough for pie, and sweet enough without honey.

SNOW ICE CREAM

(An Unusual Treat)

In top of large double boiler (or make a large one by setting a kettle or large pyrex bowl in a large kettle with water in it):

> 1 cup of cold water
> 1 tablespoon gelatin

Turn on burner and let gelatin melt in. Add:

> 1½ cups of turbinado sugar. Let melt in.

In blender:

> 6 eggs, blend and slowly add while running:
> 2 cups of dry milk
> 1 cup of oil (soybean is good)

This is quite thick. Add slowly to hot mixture in double boiler, stirring hard with a wire whip. As soon as it's hot and very smooth, take off hot water at once. Let get hot, but do not overcook. Add about 2 tablespoons vanilla and about ¼ teaspoon almond (just a touch, not too much).

Let cool. Then add snow until it's thick as ice cream. The colder it is, of course, the thicker and richer you will have it. Snow can be added while it is still warm, if they absolutely can't wait. But it will be thinner and less rich. This makes about a gallon finished product—enough for 6 people to make pigs of themselves, or enough for a crowd for dessert.

FUDGEMELLOS

Everything stays uncooked in this concoction.
>   1 cup hot water
>   2 tablespoons plain gelatin

Blend up until white and fluffed; add
>   2 egg yolks
>   ½ cup honey
>   5 tablespoons carob
>   ⅓ cup oil
>   ½ cup chopped nuts

Beat the egg whites stiff in a bowl and pour blender mixture over, folding in well. Pour into pan, chill until very stiff. Cut into squares. Can be rolled in chopped nuts and kept at room temperature for short intervals.